What's in Your Cosmetics?

A complete
consumer's guide to
natural and synthetic
ingredients

D1468825

Aubrey
Hampton

Odonian Press
TUCSON, ARIZONA

Additional copies of this and other wonderful books are available from Odonian Press, Box 32375, Tucson AZ 85751 (please see the inside back cover for information on our other titles and details on ordering). To order by credit card, or for information on quantity discounts, call us at 520 296 4056 or 800 REAL STORY, or fax us at 520 296 0936. Distribution to the book trade is through Publishers Group West, Box 8843, Emeryville CA 94662, 510 658 3453 (toll-free: 800 788 3123).

Disclaimer

No part of this book is intended for the treatment of disease, and neither the author nor the publisher assumes any liability for such use. Readers with skin conditions or other ailments should seek competent medical advice. The descriptions herein of products or substances are for educational purposes only and are not intended as recommendations by the author or publisher. The use of any product or substance discussed in this book rests on the judgement of the reader.

Trademark notice

Because a major purpose of this book is to describe and comment on various cosmetic ingredients, some such products are identified by their tradenames. In most—if not all—cases, these designations are claimed as legally protected trademarks by the companies that make the products.

It is not our intent to use any of these names generically, and the reader is cautioned to investigate a claimed trademark before using it for any purpose except to refer to the product to which it is attached.

Library of Congress Cataloging-in-Publication Data

Hampton, Aubrey, 1934–

    What's in your cosmetics? : a complete consumer's guide to natural and synthetic ingredients / Aubrey Hampton
      p.   cm.
    ISBN 1-878825-45-3
    1. Cosmetics—Composition—Dictionaries   I. Title
RA1270.C65H36   1995   95-11514
646.7'2—dc20   CIP

To the memory of my mother.
Margarette Cherie. the root woman.
who taught me how to do what I do.

to my father. Hugh Hampton. the organic farmer.
who taught me that humans and animals
share the earth

and to Ms. Hamilton. the New England herbalist.
who taught me what I know about herbs.

Text, charts, diagrams and technical accuracy: Aubrey Hampton

Editing (except herb chart), inside design and page layout:
Arthur Naiman

Copyediting and proofreading (except herb chart):
Susan McCallister, Arthur Naiman

Formatting: Elizabeth D'Onofrio, Arthur Naiman, Sarah Klein

Cover illustration, design and type: Trevor Irvin (Atlanta)

Photos in Chapter 4: M. J. Wilson

Models in Chapter 4: Flori Bess (skin care and facial massage),
Kimberly Koch (hair care)

Author photo on back cover: Josef Karsh

Fonts: Basilia (text), Bauhaus (titles, headers, footers, etc.),
Optima (tables, charts, notes), Gazelle (dedication)

Printing: Michelle Selby, Jim Puzey et al.
Consolidated Printers, Berkeley CA

Series editor: Arthur Naiman

Odonian Press gets its name from Ursula Le Guin's wonderful novel *The Dispossessed* (though we have no connection with Ms. Le Guin or any of her publishers). The last story in her collection *The Wind's Twelve Quarters* also features the Odonians.

Odonian Press donates at least 10% of its aftertax income to organizations working for social justice.

Contents

A comprehensive, alphabetical guide to more
than a thousand of the natural and synthethic
ingredients used in cosmetics, and the technical
terms that describe them

An easy-to-use listing of the cosmetic and
medicinal uses of herbs

An analysis of actual labels from cosmetics,
and a comparison of the sorts of ingredients
natural and synthetic manufacturers use

Illustrated, step-by-step procedures for
effective, natural skin care, facial massage
and hair care

Introduction

People today prefer natural vitamins, foods and cosmetics because they feel better when they use them, because natural products are better for the environment, and out of nostalgia for an earlier time when these products were made in a simple manner by herbalists, farmers and craftspeople.

Unfortunately, while the word *organic* has a legal definition, the word *natural* does not. A product with "no artificial colors or preservatives" may contain many other synthetic chemicals. The only way to know is to read the label, but what do all those chemical names mean?

If the label of a shampoo lists "sodium lauryl sulfate (from coconut oil)," is it a natural product? Well, not only isn't it natural, it usually isn't even made from coconut oil (for details, look up *sodium lauryl sulfate* in Chapter 1).

This book not only tells you which ingredients are natural and which aren't, but also which ones are likely to cause allergic reactions and what effects various chemicals have on the environment—in their production, their disposal, or both. It discusses many natural ingredients that are great for your hair and skin—like Rosa Mosqueta®, horsetail, coltsfoot, white camellia oil, jojoba oil, goa, essential fatty acids and lactalbumin. It summarizes the simple lesson I've learned in more than fifty years of creating totally natural and organic products, beginning at the age of nine at my mother's side: *Natural is better.*

Aubrey Hampton

Chapter 1
An encyclopedia of ingredients and terms

In alphabetizing, we ignore spaces, hyphens and other punctuation. Numbers are alphabetized as if they were spelled out; & is alphabetized as and.

When a term appears in italics in the text of a definition, it typically means there's an entry for that term as well, either here in Chapter 1 or in the herb chart in Chapter 2. But be aware that sometimes terms are italicized for other reasons (when they're the scientific names for plants and animals, for example), and that not all terms for which there's a cross-reference are italicized.

---

abietic acid
Used in soaps as a texturizer, and in industry in plastics and paint, this chemical is derived from pine rosin. It can cause allergic reactions and pollutes marine life. It's also known as abitol and abietyl alcohol.

abrasives
The most commonly used are *calcium carbonate* (chalk) and, in toothpaste, *di-calcium phosphate dihydrate*.

absolutes
Pure *essential oils* obtained from plants (generally flowers) and used in products as natural fragrance additives.

absorption base
A mixture or compound that acts as a carrier for ingredients and increases the absorption of these

ingredients by the skin. The use of absorption bases probably goes back to the beginnings of cosmetics in ancient Egypt. One absorption base used in Germany in 1880 was a mixture of 55% *lanolin*, 34.5% water, 10% lanolin alcohol and 0.5% *essential oils*. A natural absorption base I've created and used for some time consists of *essential fatty acids (EFAs)*, *aloe vera* and *vitamins A, C* and *E*.

acacia

The use of gum from the acacia tree dates back 4,000 years to the Egyptians, who used it in cosmetics and to manufacture paints. It's used as a stabilizer in foods and in candy, and as a foam stabilizer in soft drinks. In cosmetics, it's used as a film-forming agent (in hairsprays and gels, for example). It's also known as *gum arabic* and *catechu*. Also see *gums*.

acetarsol

This chemical, used in mouthwashes, toothpaste and feminine hygiene products, can cause allergic reactions, can be toxic and has caused cancer in lab mice. It's also known as acetarsone.

acetic acid

This *organic acid* is found in *vinegar* (at a concentration of about 6%) and various fruits, as well as in human sweat. It's used in hair dyes and hand lotions and as a bleaching lotion for freckles. It can be irritating to the skin and toxic to the lungs.

acetone

This colorless, *volatile* liquid is sometimes used in *astringents*, nail polish, nail polish removers and preservatives. It's extremely toxic.

acetone chloroform

This preservative, an *alcohol* with a camphor-like odor, has acute oral toxicity. It can be absorbed into the skin and is a strong sensitizer that causes many allergic reactions. It's used in cosmetics in concentrations of up to 0.5%, but is prohibited in aerosol dispensers.

Also known as *chlorobutanol,* acetone chloroform is sold to cosmetic manufacturers as crystals under the trade names of Chloreton, Chlorbutol, Methaform and Sedaform. Labels containing this product should have a warning that reads: *Contains chlorbutol* or *Contains chlorobutanol.*

acid

A substance with a *pH* below 7.0 (which is the pH of water). A common acid used in cosmetics is *citric acid.* (Technically, acids contain hydrogen that can be replaced by metals to form *salts,* and that is capable of dissociating in an aqueous solution to form hydrogen ions.) The adjective is *acidic.* Compare *alkali.*

acid balanced

A pseudo-scientific advertising term used to sell shampoos and skin cleansers. The *pH* of hair and skin ranges from 4.5 to 5.5. The pH of an "acid balanced" product is adjusted within this range—although a product's pH generally drifts over time and changes as soon as it's used on the hair or skin.

"Acid balanced" (also called "pH balanced") products have been around for more than a decade. At this time, their use hasn't seemed to improve the hair or skin in any way. Products that are "acid balanced" use the same synthetic chemicals as those that aren't.

Unfortunately, this slogan lures consumers into a false sense of doing something natural or scientific for their hair. Don't let advertising slogans distract you from the all-important ingredients list on the label.

acid color
This large group of *inorganic* dyes includes many *FD&C* and *D&C* colors. Also see *colors.*

acid mantle
This slightly acidic mixture of *fatty acids* and perspiration on the surface of the skin protects it from bacterial growth, but there's disagreement as to whether the *pH* of the acid mantle or the *bacteriostatic* nature of the fatty acids is the reason for the protection.

acid rinse
An acid rinse is useful for removing soap films from the hair after shampooing. A solution of vinegar or lemon juice and water is a natural one.

acne
Acne is an inflammation of the *sebaceous glands* due to retained secretions. (For a good natural treatment, see *Kummerfeld's lotion.*) The best-known type is *acne vulgaris,* the pimples on the face, chest and shoulders that commonly occur in adolescence, but there are several other kinds:

Acne artificialis is caused by external irritants or drugs taken orally. *Acne atrophica* is a type of acne vulgaris in which the lesions of the pimples leave a slight amount of scarring. *Acne cachechticorum* most commonly occurs in people with anemia or some other debilitating constitutional disease. *Acne hypertrophica* leaves conspicuous pits and scars after healing.

Acne indurata involves deeply seated pimples with hard tubercular lesions that occur chiefly on the back. In *acne keratos,* inflamed horny plugs (papules) erupt from the hair follicles. *Acne punctata* appears as red papules, usually accompanied by blackheads.

   Acne pustulosa is a type of vulgaris in which pustular lesions predominate. In *acne rosacea,* congestion causes capillaries (usually around the cheeks and nose) to become dilated and on occasion broken. *Acne simplex* consists of simple, uncomplicated pimples.

additive
A substance, either natural or synthetic, that's added to a product during or after the product is made.

adermykon
This odorless *alcohol* is used as a topical *fungicide* in cosmetics in concentrations of 0.5%. Although it causes skin rashes, dry, scaly skin and allergic reactions, it's considered to be low in toxicity in animal tests.

   A white crystalline powder, adermykon is synthesized by condensing equimolar amounts of P-chlorophenol and glycidol with tertiary *amine* or *quaternary ammonium salts*. Trade names for this preservative include Chlorphenesin, Geophen and Mycil.

adipose tissue
Tissue where fat is stored, consisting of connective tissue in which the cells are distended with fat.

adulterate
To falsify or alter by combining a foreign substance with a natural one.

aerosol
The use of aerosol sprays began in the US Army. One of the earliest patents for aerosol use in cosmetics was granted to R.W. Moore in 1903 for a perfume atomizer; carbon dioxide was used as the propellant. Aerosol sprays are toxic and harmful to the environment (fluo-

rocarbons have been made illegal for this reason). And they're highly flammable. Use pump bottles instead.

aesthetician (or esthetician)
A professional who works to clean and beautify the skin. A natural aesthetician uses only natural substances and methods to care for the skin.

affinity
Chemical compatibility of two or more substances. Also, the force that unites atoms into molecules.

aging of skin
Though skin aging is thought to be a natural process, some effects aren't very natural. Dry and wrinkled skin is caused by cross-linking in the skin's dermal proteins (collagen, elastin and reticulin), but natural skin care can reduce this. See collagen.

albumin
A simple class of proteins that are soluble in water and are coagulated by heat. They're found in blood plasma (serum albumin), in egg whites (ovalbumin) and in milk (lactalbumin), as well as in vegetables and fruits.

alcohol
A group of organic hydroxyl compounds that includes ethanol, methanol and many others. However, the term alcohol is often used to refer specifically to ethanol.

alginic acid
This acid, obtained from brown algae, has been used to protect and soothe skin. Allantoin (from comfrey root) serves the same purpose and is a better natural material for cosmetic use.

alkali

A substance with a *pH* above 7.0 (which is the pH of water). The adjective is *alkaline.* Compare *acid.*

alkalizer

A substance that raises the *pH* of a substance, thereby making it more *alkaline.*

alkaloids

Alkaloids are natural *amines* (nitrogen-containing compounds) that have pharmacological properties and are generally of plant origin. They are widely distributed throughout the plant kingdom. Most alkaloids are insoluble (or only slightly soluble) in water. Their names end in -*ine.*

alkyloamides

These *fatty acids* are widely used in cosmetics for thickening, gelling, *emulsifying, emolliency,* skin and hair conditioning, foam boosting, foam stabilizing, cleansing, wetting, opacifying, lubricating, powder binding, skin protecting, fungicidal properties and superfatting. They're most commonly found in detergent formulations such as shampoos, bubble baths and liquid hand and body cleansers. Their two main drawbacks are that they can become contaminated with *nitrosamines* and that they're harmful to the environment.

There are four main groups of alkyloamides: *diethanolamides (DEA), monoethanolamides (MEA), monoisopropanolamides (MIPA)* and ethoxylated or *PEG* alkanolamides. The DEA group was discovered first, in 1937, when Kritchevsky combined one mole of fatty acid with two moles of diethanolamine. Diethanolamine has also been combined with palm oil, soya and tallow to create soaps.

Cocamide DEA is the best known of the DEA group. It's made with coconut oil, whole *coconut fatty acids* and stripped coconut fatty acids, combined with the *ammonia salts* of carboxylic acid. The mixture can vary from equal parts of DEA and cocamide to two parts cocamide to one part DEA. An equal mixture of DEA and cocamide is often used because it creates a thicker-looking product, but it's less water-soluble than the 2:1 ratio.

Lauramide DEA is produced by combining *lauric* and *myristic fatty acids* with DEA. It's believed to be the best foam booster in shampoos, bubble baths and other detergent systems.

Myristamide DEA is the least-used of the DEA group, because it's less effective in foaming and cleansing. It does, however, produce thicker products.

Oleamide DEA will not give the same foaming results as the other DEA types, but it's a good thickening agent. It also has some conditioning properties.

Isostearamide DEA is used in shampoos and for its viscosity-building properties. It can reduce the irritating effects caused by some chemicals, and it's promoted as a hair conditioning agent and a skin emollient.

Stearamide DEA, made from triple-pressed *stearic acid,* can add a white, pearl-like look to shampoos; it's also a thickening agent. It can be used as a *nonionic* emulsifier in water/oil emulsions. It will supposedly reduce tension between the oil and water phases, as well as increasing the emulsion's overall viscosity.

Linoleamide DEA is known mainly for its thickening properties. When used in *anionic* detergents, it forms a clear, thick product, like a gel.

Fatty acid monoethanolamides (MEAs) are used as foam boosters in shampoos and other cosmetics;

they can also be used as *waxes*. MEAs are less soluble in water, since they have only a single hydrophilic hydroxy group (DEA has two). The fatty *amides* in MEA are purer in composition than those of DEA, but remember that all the alkyloamides are harmful to the environment and can become contaminated with *nitrosamines*.

alkyl sulfates

Alkyl sulfates were developed in Germany when vegetable oils and fats were scarce and when detergents that would work well in hard water were needed. They're used in most shampoos today, and are often represented on labels as being natural and derived from coconut oil. They were *originally* derived from natural oils like coconut, palm kernel and soya, but today they're almost all produced from petrochemicals.

alkyltrimethylammonium bromide

The registered trade names of this preservative, which is often used in deodorants at concentrations of about 0.05% to 0.1%, are Arquad, Cetavlon, Cetab, Micol and Dodigen 5594. Supplied as crystals, this quaternary compound is toxic. It's inactive in the presence of soaps, *anionics,* nitrates, metals, proteins and blood.

allantoin

Allantoin is widely reported to have healing, soothing and anti-irritating properties. It can be extracted from *urea* (from the urine of most animals, including humans) or from herbs such as *comfrey* or uva ursi.

allergy

A hypersensitive reaction to specific substances that develops in some persons.

almond meal
This is the residue that remains after the oil has been expressed from almonds (usually only sweet almonds are used). Almond meal is excellent for exfoliation in face masks and soaps, and it also has soothing properties for the skin.

aloe vera
See the listing in the herb chart in Chapter 2.

alopecia
A deficiency of hair; baldness. Partial baldness is called *alopecia areata.*

alpha hydroxy acids
This is the chemical name for various acids that appear naturally in fruit. (See *fruit acids.*) They're used in toners, creams and masks to exfoliate (remove dead skin cells from) the skin, and they act as moisturizers as well.

Alpha hydroxy acids are high in *glycolic acid* and have become popular in cosmetics that exfoliate the skin, but they can be irritating to the skin, causing redness and rashes. (Procter & Gamble recently removed their alpha hydroxy acid products from the market due to skin irritation problems.)

Green tea has been found to reduce the irritating effects. The problem is less common in the natural fruit acids—the extracts of bilberry, black currant, apple, etc.—which are known as red fruit acids.

alterative
An herbal agent that gradually produces a change toward good health.

alum

Used in medicine, dyeing and industrial processes, this double sulfate of aluminum and potassium is also known as *aluminum sulfate.* In the cosmetic industry, it's used in antiperspirants, powders, antiseptics and detergents. It can cause allergic reactions, infection of the skin or hair follicles, and irritation of the lungs when inhaled. (For more on all this, see the next entry.)

In ancient times, *alum* was produced by burning herbs to obtain the ash, but today we know it as a naturally occurring mineral called kalunite, and as a constituent of the mineral alunite. The industrial alums are potash alum, ammonium alum, sodium alum and chrome alum (potassium chromium sulfate).

aluminum chemicals in cosmetics

Aluminum chemicals are used frequently in cosmetics. There's aluminum chlorohydrate in deodorants and antiperspirants, aluminum fluoride in toothpaste, alumina in *astringents,* and *alum* (described in the previous entry).

Some scientists believe that aluminum compounds cause Alzheimer's disease. The brains of Alzheimer's victims show a deficiency of acetylcholine, and anticholinergics (substances that work against acetylcholine) can produce a dementia-like state. Aluminum chemicals may disrupt the normal activity of acetylcholine. If this is true, aluminum chemicals in cosmetics should be considered dangerous.

aluminum sulfate

See *alum.*

ambergris

This secretion from the intestinal tract of the sperm whale has been used as a *fixative* in fragrances.

Because whales are endangered species, use of natural ambergris is prohibited by law in the US.

amides
Derivatives of carboxylic acid, amides are solids with low melting points. They're stable, weakly acidic and soluble in hydroxylic solvents like water and alcohol.

One popular amide, *cocamide DEA,* combines coconut fatty acid with the ammonium salts of carboxylic acid. This produces a thicker appearance and reduces the stinging effect on the eyes (though not very effectively).

Amides also improve sudsing action, and are sometimes combined with soap bark *(quillaya bark),* which is very cleansing but has a low suds factor on its own. For this and other reasons, amides are often used in soaps and shampoos. Also see *alkyloamides.*

amines
Amines (also known as acyl glutamates) are *organic* nitrogen compounds that are formed by combining *ammonia* molecules with metal ions such as calcium, strontium and barium. As *amino acids, alkaloids* and vitamins, they play a prominent role in biochemical systems and are present in substances as varied as adrenaline, thiamine and novacaine. Amines are used in shampoos to supposedly reduce the stinging effect on the eyes.

amino acids
These natural acids contain *amine* chemical groups, and link together to form *polypeptides* and proteins. *Essential amino acids* are ones that can't be manufactured by the body.

Human hair is made up of eighteen amino acids; amine links between them form large, condensed, *polymeric* structures. Because the sulfur-containing amino acids *cysteine* and methionine are essential to protein metabolism, some of the better hair- and skin-care products contain them. For more details, see the hair care section in Chapter 4.

aminophenol

This amino-type permanent hair dye has been in use since 1883. It's used to produce medium brown, orange-red and blond shades, and is toxic.

ammonia

This familiar compound, made from the elements nitrogen and hydrogen, is formed when organic material decomposes. It can easily be detected by its strong, irritating odor. It's a primary irritant and should be avoided.

Ammonia has a wide range of industrial uses. For example, it's used in the production of nitric acid, ammonium salts, the sulfates (used in many shampoo ingredients), nitrate (used as a preservative in meats and in shampoos), carbonate and chloride, and in the synthesis of hundreds of compounds, including drugs, plastics, hair dyes and permanent wave solutions.

ammoniated mercury

See *mercury and its compounds.*

ammonium carbonate

This chemical, which is used as a *pH* adjuster in many permanent wave preparations, can sensitize the face, scalp, hands and cause *contact dermatitis.*

18

ammonium hydroxide
Used in hair waving solutions, hair straighteners and detergents, this highly caustic chemical can irritate the mucous membranes and even burn the skin. It's also harmful to the environment.

amphoteric surfactants
Amphoterics (also known as *surface-active* agents) possess both a positive and negative electrical charge, and are capable of reacting as either an *acid* or an alkali, depending on the rest of the formula. They're promoted to cosmetic manufacturers (and thus indirectly to consumers) as being milder and better than the *alkyl sulfate* detergents discussed above. Many shampoo ingredients combine an alkyl sulfate detergent and an amphoteric surfactant; cocoamide betaine is one example. Also see *alkyloamides*.

amyl acetate
This toxic solvent, used in nail polish, acts as a central nervous system depressant and skin irritant. Inhalation of its vapors is harmful to the respiratory system.

amyl dimethyl PABA
This combination of *PABA ester* and amyl alcohol is used in sunscreens. It can cause *eczema* and allergic *dermatitis*. Instead, look for natural food-grade PABA in your sunscreens; it's compounded in vegetable glycerine and gives fewer allergic reactions.

analgesic
A substance that relieves or eliminates pain. Also called an *anodyne*. Compare *anesthetic*.

anesthetic
A substance that reduces or eliminates sensation, including pain. Compare *analgesic* and *anodyne*.

angelica *(Archangelica officinalis)*
For thousands of years, the Chinese have been using
the roots, leaves and seeds of ten angelica species to
make dang-gui, a treatment for female ailments.
When applied as a skin tonic or lotion, angelica has a
soothing effect on the nerves of the skin. It's also used
as a fragrance by perfumers.

Angelica contains bergapten and xanthotoxin and,
like bergamot, it can be *phototoxic;* however, the
seed oil is not phototoxic. Angelica has *antibacterial*
properties, and is used as a treatment for *psoriasis.*
See *ching-shang.*

anhydrous
This term indicates that a substance is water-free
(e.g., anhydrous lanolin).

aniline dyes
Discovered in Germany in 1873, aniline dyes are
made from *coal tar,* a suspected human carcinogen.
They're used in hair dyes. Also see *colors.*

anionic
Having a negative electrical charge. Compare *cationic*
and *nonionic.*

anionic surfactants
These synthetic, *surface-active* agents form the base
detergent in most shampoos, including those that are
called "natural." They're inexpensive for manufacturers but hard on consumers' hair. (*Anionic* refers to
their negative electrical charge.)

A serious problem with anionic surfactants is that
they may be contaminated with NDLA (N-nitrosodiethanolamine), one of the *nitrosamines* and a potent
carcinogen (according to a 1977 FDA report). Sham-

pooing the hair with a product contaminated with NDLA can lead to its absorption into the body at levels much higher than eating nitrite-contaminated foods. Thus all the following anionic surfactants should be avoided:

> *Sodium lauryl sulfate, TEA-lauryl sulfate,* ammonium lauryl sulfate, *sodium laureth sulfate,* TEA laureth sulfate, ammonium laureth sulfate, lauroyl sarcosine, cocoyl sarcosine, sodium lauroyl sarcosinate, sodium cocoyl sarcosinate, potassium coco-hydrolyzed animal protein, disodium oleamide sulfosuccinate, sodium dioctyl sulfosuccinate, sodium methyl oleoyl sulfate and sodium lauryl isoethionate.

anodyne
A substance that relieves or eliminates pain. Also called an *analgesic.* Compare *anesthetic.*

anthelmintic
A substance that destroys or expels intestinal parasites. Also called a *vermifuge.*

anthraquinone dye
See *colors.*

antibacterial
This term, which means *hostile to bacteria,* differs slightly but significantly from *bacteriostatic,* which refers to substances that create an environment in which bacteria don't want to live. Natural substances, such as herbal *essential oils,* tend to be bacteriostatic. Antibacterials are also known as *bactericides.*

anticoagulant
A substance that reduces or prevents clotting of the blood. Opposite of *coagulant.*

anticonvulsive
A substance that relieves or prevents convulsions.

antidandruff shampoo
Most antidandruff shampoos contain *colloidal sulfur, zinc pyrrithione, salicylic acid* or *resorcinol,* which are mixed into the usual harsh synthetic detergent base and preserved with the *parabens.* There are, however, natural dandruff treatments, such as selenium sulfide, *jojoba oil, amino acids,* indigofera, *quillaya bark* and *aloe vera.* Look for a mild shampoo that won't be irritating to a dandruff-prone scalp. See the natural hair care section in Chapter 4.

anti-emetic
A substance that relieves vomiting.

anti-inflammatory
A substance that reduces inflammation. Also called an *antiphlogistic.*

antioxidants
These substances, which have received much publicity in recent years as potential life-extenders, prevent the too-rapid *oxidation* of nutrients, and counter the destructive effects of free radicals (chemically reactive molecules) in the body. Antioxidants can be natural or synthetic, and there are several types.

Antioxidant vitamins are A, E, C complex (including *ascorbic acid,* rutin, bioflavonoids and hesperidin), B complex (including thiamine, niacin, *pantothenic acid,* pyridoxine, *PABA, inositol* and choline). Antioxidant minerals include selenium and *zinc.* Antioxidant enzymes, produced by the body, are superoxide dismutase (SOD) and glutathione peroxidase. *Cysteine* is an antioxidant *amino acid.* There are even a couple of antioxidant synthetic food additives: *BHA* and *BHT*.

Natural antioxidants like vitamins A, C and E can be used to preserve cosmetics, but more usually BHA or BHT are used.

antiparalytic
A substance that relieves paralysis.

antiperiodic
In herbology, a substance that acts against recurring diseases like intermittent fevers.

antiperspirant
A substance or product that inhibits or prevents perspiration. Antiperspirants block the pores of the skin and can cause allergic reactions. Also see *deodorant*.

antiphlogistic
In herbology, a substance that reduces inflammation. Also called an *anti-inflammatory*.

antipruritic
A substance that relieves itching.

antipyretic
A substance that relieves rheumatism and reduces or prevents fever.

antiscorbutic
A substance that, because it contains *vitamin C*, cures or prevents scurvy.

antiseptic
A substance that destroys or inhibits the growth of bacteria and other microorganisms *(sepsis* means putrefaction or decay). Many herbs have natural anti-

septic action, which is preferable to the harsher synthetic antiseptics. See Chapter 2 for details.

antispasmodic
A substance that relieves or reduces spasms.

antitussive
A substance that relieves or inhibits coughing.

aperient
A substance that relieves constipation.

aphrodisiac
A substance that arouses sexual desire.

aqueous
Containing, or relating to, water.

aromatherapy
This is the art of using *essential oils* from roots, barks and herbs for treating the skin and body. Each herb has various therapeutic, vitalizing effects on the dermis and subcutaneous tissues to varying degrees, whether it's inhaled, steamed or massaged into the body.

Essential oils can be powerful therapeutic agents and should be used in tiny amounts in cosmetic formulas. By using them, we can create cosmetics that are as natural as possible.

aromatic
In herbology, a substance with an agreeable odor or stimulating qualities.

ascorbic acid
Also known as *vitamin C,* this *organic* acid occurs naturally in many plants, especially citrus fruits. Due to its *antioxidant* qualities, it can be used as a preservative in food and cosmetics. Large amounts are needed

to preserve some cosmetics, but it works well when combined with the antioxidant vitamins A and E.

The fat-soluble form of vitamin C, ascorbyl palmitate, works better in emulsions and cosmetic oils than ascorbic acid, which is water-soluble. Combining the two forms protects both the water phase and oil phase of a cosmetic from microorganisms. Both are supplied as a white powder, and are completely nontoxic; topical use will not irritate the skin.

asteatosis
A deficiency or absence of *sebaceous* secretions.

astragulus *(Astragulus hoantchy)*
The sweet-tasting root of this Chinese herb is known as huang-chi and is used as an energy *tonic, diuretic* and *antipyretic.* Though it has little use in cosmetics, it can be utilized as an *astringent.*

astringent
Because astringents cause organic tissues to contract, they're used to clean the skin of oils and other substances on its surface. They can be synthetic or natural (natural astringents include *witch hazel, benzoin* gum extract and other *tonic* herbs). The use of a natural herbal astringent is recommended after the skin is thoroughly cleansed, to remove soap films and cellular debris.

athlete's foot
A fungus infection of the foot.

atractylodes *(Atractylodes ovata)*
The rhizome of this herb, known in China as tsang-chu, is used as an aromatic and a *tonic,* for intestinal

problems and for pigmentation problems on the skin. See *tang-kuei.*

azine

This acid-quinonoid type of synthetic color is toxic and harmful to the environment. Also see *colors.*

azo colors *or* dyes

The largest group of *coal tar* colors, azo colors are toxic, harmful to the environment, and may be carcinogenic. Also see *colors.*

azulene

This *anti-inflammatory* agent is extracted from the camomile flower and used for its soothing qualities. Azulene from Moroccan blue camomile is superior to that from Hungarian blue camomile.

baby products

Hair, skin and body care products specifically made for babies include baby oil, shampoo, talcum powder, soap and lotion. Only a few natural brands are available and it's necessary to carefully choose among them based on their labels.

For example, baby shampoos that claim to prevent "tears" when the soap gets in the child's eyes should be avoided, because they contain chemicals that anesthetize the eyes and can be dangerous. Tearing is an important natural function and shouldn't be prevented.

Synthetic chemicals are even more toxic for small people than adults, so natural ingredients are very important here. One good natural ingredient to look for is *evening primrose oil,* which is an effective treatment for *eczema.* Read the labels!

bactericide
An *antibacterial* agent.

bacteriostatic
See *antibacterial*.

baking soda
Also known as sodium bicarbonate, baking soda relieves burns, itching, urticarial lesions and insect bites. It's often used in bath powders to help cleanse oily skin, and is a common component of many home-made cosmetics and food preparations. It's an excellent tooth powder on its own, and when combined with *aloe vera* gel, it's the best toothpaste you can use.

balneotherapy
The scientific medical study of bathing and its effects on the human body.

balsams
These healing or soothing agents contain relatively large amounts of cinnamic or *benzoic acid.* While benzoic acid is toxic in its synthetic versions and in tinctures like *sodium benzoate* (as was first pointed out by Adelle Davis and others), *benzoin gum* and other balsams that contain benzoates aren't toxic—in fact, they're helpful. Typical balsams are *balsam of Peru, balsam tolu, storax* and *benzoin.* For more on them, see their entries in the herb chart in Chapter 2.

barium sulfide
A toxic and caustic chemical in many cosmetic preparations, especially hair relaxers.

barrier creams
These are applied to the skin to provide a protective coating against chemical irritants.

basal layer
The layer of skin at the base of the *epidermis* (closest to the *dermis).*

bayberry wax
See *waxes.*

bee pollen
This natural substance is high in *pantothenic acid,* and European research suggests it may be helpful in combating the effects of radiation exposure. However, it's not particularly valuable as a *topical.*

beeswax
This natural substance is obtained from the honeycomb of the honeybee, *Apis mellifera,* as well as other Apis species. Both yellow beeswax and white beeswax are used as thickeners, *emulsifiers* or stiffening agents in ointments, cold creams, *emollient* creams, lotions, lipsticks, hair dressings, suppositories and other cosmetics. *Vegans* will want to avoid products with beeswax. Also see *waxes.*

beet powder
This natural, nontoxic color is made from powdered beet root and is sometimes used in cosmetics.

behenic acid
This crystalline mixture of *fatty acids* from seeds (such as peanuts) is used as an opacifier in cosmetics.

bentonite
This soft, moisture-absorbing, clay mineral, often of volcanic origin, contains *montmorillonite* as its essential mineral. Used as a suspending agent, *emulsifier,* thickener, binder and absorbent, and in mask products, it may be drying to the skin. It's called *bentonite*

because it originally came from Benton, Montana. Also see *clay* and *kaolin.*

benzaldehyde

This synthetic chemical is used as an artificial almond oil, and also as a preservative and solvent. It's irritating to the eyes, skin and mucous membranes.

benzalkonium chloride

This quaternary *(cationic)* compound has been shown to be highly toxic and shouldn't be inhaled. It's also a primary skin irritant and is a common source of eye irritations.

Benzalkonium chloride is used in hair conditioners and conditioning shampoos (the cationic types), cream rinses and deodorants, in concentrations of 0.1% to 0.5%; it's also used as an antiseptic and a germicide. It's inactive when used with *anionics,* soaps, proteins, plastics, rubber, citrates, metals and nitrates. Some trade names of this preservative are Zephirol, Roccal, Dodigen 226 and Barquat MB-50.

benzene

This petrochemical, which is used as a solvent and manufacturing agent in cosmetics, can cause depression, convulsions, coma and death; prolonged exposure is suspected of causing leukemia. Benzene vapors can be absorbed through the skin and cause irritation. Benzene should be avoided.

benzethonium chloride

This common ingredient in many feminine hygiene products can sensitize and irritate the skin, possibly leading to allergic dermatitis. It's also used as a preservative.

benzoic acid

This *organic acid,* derived from *benzoin gum,* is used as a preservative in some cosmetics, typically at concentrations of 0.1%−0.2% (with a maximum concentration of 0.5%). It's only effective at low *pHs:* for example, at pH 2, it's 99% effective; pH 3, 94%; at pH 4, 60%; at pH 5, 13%; and it's hardly effective at all above pH 5. For this reason, it won't work in most shampoo formulas.

Although it's found in nature in many berries, roots and herbs, benzoic acid is acutely toxic both orally and topically (a toxic dose on the skin is 6 mg/kg). In spite of that, it's used as a preservative in foods (especially beverages) and in pharmaceuticals.

The suggested oral intake is up to 5 mg/kg per day. Lab animals have been murdered by feeding them 80 mg/kg for a three-month period, or 40 mg/kg for seventeen months. It's also stunted the growth of mice and rats.

Benzoic acid was first described by H. Fleck in 1875, but it was probably used in the form of the herb *benzoin* before that. Supplied in tablet form or as a white powder, it's soluble in water (at 20° C) and in alcohol.

benzoin, benzoin gum

A *balsamic resin* found in various species of an Asian tree called the *storax* (or styrax), benzoin gum is formed when the bark is incised; the exuded resin, which hardens on exposure to air and sunlight, is then collected. Benzoin, especially Siam benzoin, has *antioxidative* properties and the natural extract is used in some cosmetics, though more often a synthetic version, such as *sodium benzoate,* is used.

benzyl alcohol
This natural, aromatic *alcohol* is found in many herbs, including balsam Peru, canaga oil, cassie absolute, castoreum, cherry laurel leaves, jasmine and storax. It's used in injectable drugs, ophthalmic products and oral liquids, as a solvent in cosmetics and perfumes, and as a preservative in hair dyes.

In oral products, benzyl alcohol is used at concentrations between 0.5% and 2%, and in cosmetics at 1% to 3%. It has a high percutaneous toxicity and it can cause allergic reactions. It's also known as benzenemethanol, phenylcarbinol and phenylmethanol.

benzyl carbinol
This preservative is a natural *alcohol* found in *essential oils* such as rose, hyacinth and aleppo pine. It's toxic internally at 1.79 g/kg and on the skin at 5–10 ml/kg; it irritates human eyes at concentrations of 0.75%. It's also known as phenethyl alcohol.

beta carotene
See *carotenoids*.

betaine
An *alkaloid* present in beets.

BHA and BHT
BHA (butylated hydroxyanisole) and BHT (butylated hydroxytoluene) are synthetic *antioxidants* approved for use in food and cosmetics. Also see *antioxidants*.

biochemistry
The study of the chemical compounds and processes that occur in living plants and animals.

biodegradable
This term refers to substances that can be broken down by natural processes into chemical components that can reenter the natural world without changing it. Many "biodegradable" household cleaners, cosmetics and other products are far less biodegradable than their labeling would lead you to believe, thanks to various preservatives and other chemicals used in them. Read the label to be sure the product is natural.

biotin
One of the B vitamins that helps dermatitis and hair loss. Also see *vitamin B complex.*

bisulfites *and* sulfites
These *inorganic acids* are toxic, causing headaches, nausea or diarrhea at doses lower than 50 mg/kg of body weight. Lab animals fed 0.5%–2% bisulfite in food showed injuries to the nervous system within a year; those fed 0.25% had diarrhea but no other toxic effects. Although neither human nor animal tests show these preservatives to be safe, they're used at concentrations of 0.2% in cosmetics and at 1%–2% as preservatives and disinfectants in foods (especially wines).

The sulfites are supplied as white powders and the bisulfites as clear to semi-clear solutions (which aren't stable). Some of the sulfites are also soluble in water.

bitter
Bitterness in an herb promotes the production of saliva and gastric juices, thereby increasing appetite and digestion.

blackhead
This skin blemish results from an oily secretion of *sebum* and dead cells that clogs the hair follicle; the

plug darkens when it comes into contact with the air. Blackheads differ from *whiteheads* in that the follicle remains open to the air; whiteheads are covered with a layer of skin and are thus more likely to become infected. Deep cleansing of the skin can help prevent blackheads. Also see *acne*.

blue light
A therapeutic lamp used to soothe the nerves and also to heal and disinfect skin tissue.

bond
A bond is a molecular linkage between two different atoms or radicals of a chemical compound, usually altered by the transfer of one or more electrons from one atom to another. In chemical formulas, a bond is represented by a dot or line between atoms.

borates
This generic term refers to *salts* related to boric oxide or orthoboric acid. See *borax* and *boric acid* for examples.

borax
This naturally occurring mineral (also known as pyroborate, diborate or sodium borate) is used to manufacture glass, ceramic glazes, enamels, water-softening agents, flame-proofing materials, preservatives and fluxes. It may be harmful if breathed into the lungs during manufacturing or processing.

In cosmetics, borax is used as an *emulsifier*. When combined with *beeswax* in a cream, it usually makes up about 6% of the weight of the wax. As the concentration of borax increases, the cream stiffens.

boric acid

Boric acid, also known as acidum boricum or ortho-boric acid, is used widely as an eyewash. An odorless, white, crystalline powder, it can be used around windows and doors as a bug repellent. It shouldn't be used in baby cosmetics or baby powder, since it's toxic at doses of 1–3 g for babies, 5 g for children and 15–20 g for adults.

boron

This mineral makes up 0.001% of the earth's crust and is found at concentrations of a few parts per million in sea water. In small amounts, it's vital to all forms of plant life, but in large amounts, it's toxic. There are many *organic* compounds of boron, including *boric acid.*

botanical

Any substance obtained from plants which has medicinial or similar uses.

bran

See *wheat bran.*

brewer's yeast

High in protein and all the B vitamins, this powder is sometimes added to cosmetics for its nutritional value. Also see *vitamin B complex.*

bromelain

This enzyme, extracted from pineapple juice, hydrolyzes proteins. It's used in cosmetics as a texturizer and keratolytic.

bromochlorophene

This *phenolic compound* is acutely toxic when taken orally.

bronopol
This toxic *alcohol* is used in fabric softeners and detergents, in pharmaceutical products, and in face creams, shampoos, hair dressings, mascaras and bath oils at concentrations of 0.01% to 0.1%. Supplied as a white crystalline powder, it causes skin irritation at concentrations of 0.25%.

butyl acetate
This toxic solvent is used in nail polishes and in many other products.

butylene glycol
This thick liquid, used in hair rinses and conditioners, causes many allergic reactions and is harmful to the environment.

butyl stearate
This synthetic chemical is found in face creams and other facial care products. It's a possible allergen and has caused acne cosmetica (acne caused by cosmetics).

butyrolactone
This very toxic, synthetic chemical is used as a solvent for *resins* in cosmetics, especially nail polish removers.

C.
Abbreviation for Celsius, or Centigrade, the temperature scale (used virtually everywhere in the world except the U.S.) in which water freezes at 0° and boils at 100°. Compare *F.*

calamine
This pink powder, made of *zinc oxide* with a small amount of ferric oxide (an *inorganic salt),* is used in lotions, ointments and liniments. It's a traditional mixture that is soothing and healing to the skin, especially

for itchy rashes such as poison ivy. Though calamine is natural, some formulas contain *phenol,* which may cause phenol poisoning when applied to the skin. A mixture of natural calamine with *aloe vera* is a good skin treatment for burns, rashes and insect bites.

calcium
Various forms of this mineral, which makes up 3.64% of the earth's crust, are used as "whiteners" and in toothpastes as a polishing agent. Recently, calcium supplements have been recognized as preventive nutrition for osteoporosis, and women have been advised to get 1000–1500 mg daily. Check the label of calcium supplements for the salt content; sodium compounds of calcium are often used because they're less expensive (one-fifth to one-sixth the price).

calcium acetate
This calcium *salt* of *acetic acid* is a synthetic chemical that's used in cosmetics as an *emulsifier* and thickener. It can cause allergic reactions.

calcium alginate
This nontoxic calcium *salt* of *alginic acid* is used in many food products and as a binding and disintegrating agent in tablets. It's also used as a film-former in peel-off masks, a suspending and thickening agent in cosmetic gels, lotions and creams, and as a stabilizer for oil-in-water *emulsions.* (Alginates are *hydrophilic* colloidal substances extracted from certain brown algae, particularly macrocystic, laminaria and ascophyllum.)

calcium carbonate
This naturally occurring *salt* is found in limestone, chalk and marble. It's used as a pigment and pigment

extender in *dentifrices* and antacids, and in making lime and whiting. It has no known toxicity.

calcium chloride
Commonly used in road salt and antifreeze, this calcium *salt* is used in cosmetics as an *emulsifier* and texturizer. Taken internally, it can cause constipation and stomach problems, and it can cause lung difficulties if inhaled during manufacturing or processing, but its toxicity in cosmetics is not known.

calcium hydroxide
Also known as hydrated lime or limewater, this caustic substance is used as an *alkalizer* and a preservative in *depilatories,* and as a topical *astringent.* It can cause burns to the skin and eyes, and ingesting it can burn the throat and esophagus—and even cause death from shock and asphyxia due to swelling of the voice box. Avoid this chemical and keep it away from children.

calcium silicate
This anticaking agent is used in heavy manufacturing and also in cosmetics like face powders as a coloring agent. It can cause allergic reactions to the skin and may irritate lungs if inhaled.

calcium sulfate
This mineral, mined in New York, Michigan, Texas, Iowa and Ohio, is used in cement and to reduce the alkalinity of soil. Calcium sulfate is also used to make gypsum and asbestos ($CaMg_3CSiO_3$). These products are carcinogens when breathed or absorbed into the body.

calmative
Any substance that has a calming or tranquilizing effect.

cancer
See *carcinogenicity in cosmetics.*

candelilla wax
This herbal wax, obtained from various *Euphorbia-ceae* species, is used in lipsticks, in creams and as a substitute for rubber. It can be used with other waxes to harden them. Also see *waxes.*

candida albicans
The common cause of yeast infections, this fungus is usually present in the body in small amounts, but when it overgrows, it can dominate other microorganisms. This imbalance leads to a variety of symptoms: exhaustion, intestinal gas, sugar craving, alternating constipation and diarrhea, mood swings, depression, irritation, memory loss, dizziness, muscle aches, mysterious weight gain, vaginal or prostate itch. Acidophilus tablets are a natural treatment, and topically applied *evening primrose oil* (EPO) and EPO cream can also help. Also see *evening primrose oil.*

canthanaxin
This reddish *carotenoid* is found in some mushrooms and shellfish; it's also the chemical that makes flamingos pink. Taken in large quantities, it will have the same effect on you, coloring your skin a reddish bronze. What it does to the rest of you while it's doing that is unknown. We don't recommend it—too much sun is not good for your skin, but canthanaxin is not a safe alternative. Also see *colors.*

capric acid
This crystalline *fatty acid* with a low boiling point is used in cosmetics as a flavoring and an *aromatic*. It

has no known toxicity. It gets its name from its goat-like odor *(caper* is Latin for *goat)*.

capsicum oleoresin
This resinous *essential oil* from the pepper family is used in hair tonics to stimulate the scalp. It's said to promote hair growth, but it may cause allergic reactions in some people.

captan
This *phenolic* compound is used in soaps and shampoos at concentrations of 0.5%, and as an agricultural *fungicide*. We must regard this product as toxic due to the presence of phenol.

Captan is a phthalimid derivative sold under the trade names Vancid 89 RE and Advacide TMP. Phthaleins are formed by treating phthalic anhydride with phenols.

caramel
A concentrated solution of heated sugar or glucose, caramel is used in cosmetics as a color, in skin lotions as a soothing agent, and in food as a flavoring and coloring agent. The FDA ruled that caramel is *GRAS* (generally recognized as safe) in 1981. Also see *colors*.

carbon
See *organic*.

Carbomer 934, 940, 941, 960 and 961
This synthetic *emulsifier* and thickener is used in many cosmetics and toothpastes, as well as in industrial goods. It has a very acidic *pH* in a 1% water solution, and is an allergen that can cause eye irritation. It should be avoided.

carboxymethyl hydroethyl cellulose

This sodium *salt* of an ethylene *glycol* ether of cellulose gum is used as an *emulsifier,* foaming agent and stabilizer in cosmetics. It causes allergic reactions.

carcinogenic

Cancer-causing.

carcinogenicity in cosmetics

Not only synthetic chemicals but natural substances can be carcinogenic. One such group of natural substances are the *nitrosamines,* known carcinogens that are produced when chemicals called nitrites combine with *amines.*

This can occur in preserved pork products because of the addition of sodium nitrite (which is put in to prevent the growth of the botulism-causing organism *Clostridium botulinum),* but the bacteria normally found in salivary plaque and in the gastrointestinal tract also synthesize nitrites. These nitrites combine with secondary amines in the stomach to form alkyl-nitrosamines, which are active carcinogens. *Ascorbic acid (vitamin C)* competes with secondary amines for the nitrite and thereby reduces the amount of nitrosamine.

Nitrites are also detectable in some cosmetic chemicals and can be absorbed into the body. One potent carcinogen found in cosmetics is N-nitrosodiethanolamine (NDELA), a combination of triethanolamine (TEA) or diethanolamine (DEA) and a nitrosating agent. NDELA has been found in many cosmetics, from face creams to shampoos.

More nitrites can be absorbed into the bloodstream from using certain cosmetics than from eating nitrites that have been added to food. Prudent individuals avoid synthetic chemicals as much as possible, and regard cosmetics not simply as innocuous substances applied to the skin and the hair, but as an added burden to our environment and to our own bodies.

cardiac
Relating to the heart.

carminative
A substance that relieves gas from the intestine.

carmine
This natural red color comes from the dried female *cochineal* beetle. It's sometimes used to color lip gloss, lipsticks and other cosmetics.

carnauba wax
See *waxes*.

carotenoids
Beta carotene is the most common of these orange or red compounds that occur in plants and in the bodies of plant-eating animals. They're *antioxidants* and precursors to vitamin A. Also see the entry for *vitamin A* in this chapter and *carrot oil* in Chapter 2.

carvacrol
This *phenolic compound,* used in cosmetics at 0.1% concentrations, is toxic.

casein
A protein specific to the milk of mammals.

castile soap
Originally prepared from olive oil in much the same manner that soap is made from coconut oil, *castile* now simply refers to any very mild soap. But the finest grade of castile soap is still made from olive oil.

catalyst
A substance that increases the speed of a chemical reaction, or that causes an intended chemical change.

cataplasm
Another name for a poultice.

catechu
Another name for *acacia*.

cationic
Having a positive electrical charge. Compare *anionic* and *nonionic*.

cationic surfactant
A *surface-active* agent (like *quaternary ammonium salts*) whose ions are positively charged in an aqueous solution. Also see *anionic surfactants* and *amphoteric surfactants*.

CA 24 (chloroacetamide)
This chemical, also known as acidamide, is used as an antimicrobial in shampoos and bath lotions at concentrations of up to 0.3%. Its activity is increased by the presence of *sodium lauryl sulfate* and sodium laureth sulfate.

Humans have had allergic reactions to a 0.1% water solution of it within 24, 48 or 72 hours of use. The European Economic Community requires a label warning that reads: *Contains chloroacetamide.*

CA 24 is synthesized from ethyl chololacetate and *ammonia*. It contains 70% chloroacetamide and 30% *sodium benzoate*.

celandine
One of the herbs traditionally used for the bleaching of hair. It has no known toxicity but may cause allergic reactions in some people.

cellular extracts
Various extracts from the organs or tissues of animals (usually cows or sheep) are put into facial moisturizing creams with the claims that they'll encourage rapid healing of tissue and stimulate the growth of new healthy skin cells. They probably don't work, and herbal extracts are safer and better.

cellulose gums
Cellulose is the fiber in the cell walls of all plants. Gum made from it is used as an *emulsifier,* stabilizer and binder in cosmetics. There is no known toxicity, but inhaling the powder during manufacturing or processing can be harmful to the lungs, and allergic reactions are possible. Cellulose gum is also known as sodium carboxymethyl cellulose. Also see *gums.*

ceresin wax
See *waxes.*

certified colors
Although the FDA certifies *coal tar* or petrochemical colors as safe for use (except as hair dyes), various colors have been found to cause cancer. Since hair dyes are exempt from even this simple "certification," it's dangerous to use them. The cost to the manufacturer of getting a coal tar or petrochemical color certified is about 25¢ a pound. Also see *colors* and *hair coloring.*

cetalkonium chloride
This *quaternary ammonium salt*, used as an antiseptic and preservative, is a toxic synthetic chemical.

ceteareth-3
This polyethylene glycol of cetearyl glycol, used in cosmetics as an *emulsifier* and *emollient*, dries out the skin and causes many allergic reactions.

cetearyl alcohol
This mixture of *cetyl alcohol* and *stearyl alcohol* may be natural or synthetic. It's used as an *emollient*, *emulsifier*, thickener and carrying agent for other ingredients. Also see *fatty alcohols*.

cetyl alcohol
This solid *fatty alcohol* is used in cosmetics as an *emollient, emulsifier*, thickener and carrying agent for other ingredients. It can be synthetic or natural (obtained from coconut oil). If natural, the label should say *coconut fatty alcohol* or *natural cetyl alcohol*, but labels often aren't specific.

cetyl lactate, myristate, palmitate and stearate
These *esters* of *cetyl alcohol* and *lactic acid, myristic acid, palmitic acid* and *stearic acid*, used as *emollients* and texturizers in cosmetics, may be natural or synthetic.

chalk
Soft limestone of marine origin. Also see *calcium carbonate*.

cheilitis
This form of dermatitis involves cracking and drying of the lips. It's caused by lipstick, primarily ones containing large amounts of synthetic dyes (particularly

eosin dyes, which stain the lips), synthetic perfumes or other allergenic substances. Natural lip balms like almond or *jojoba oil,* or jojoba butter, can help.

chih-ko *(Citrus kotokan)*
The ripe fruit of this Chinese citrus is used for stomach problems. It's also used in Chinese herbal formulas for skin problems like acne. Also see *ching-shang.*

Chinese herb use
Herbs aren't used in cosmetics in China as much as they are in Europe and the US. Even *royal jelly, bee pollen* and ginseng, which you find in many cosmetics in health food stores in the US, are used as medicines in China.

ching-shang-fang-feng-tang
This herbal mixture, known in China as the *Siler* Combination for the Skin, is a classic Chinese treatment for acne, eczema, acne rosacea and various skin problems. It can be taken as a tea and also used as a face *tonic,* applied twice a day to affected areas.

Ching-shang-fang-feng-tang is made from one-half ounce each of *angelica, chih-ko, cnidium, coptis, forsythia, gardenia, licorice, mentha, platycodon, schizonepeta, scute* and *siler.* To this mixture add one gram of *coix* seeds. I usually also add half a gram of *rhubarb* and a pinch of *alum.* The herbs can be obtained at a Chinese herb shop. Note: Chinese herbal tonics should come to no more than a total weight of 16 ounces unless otherwise stated.

Even if you don't have skin problems, ching-shang-fang-feng-tang is excellent for the tone of the skin, which it leaves smooth and soft. Also see *acne.*

chlorobutanol
Another name for *acetone chloroform.*

chlorophene
This *phenolic compound,* used in cosmetics at concentrations of 0.2%, has a very limited antimicrobial activity. Due to the presence of phenolic compounds, it should be regarded as toxic.

Chlorophene is incompatible with *nonionics, quaternary* compounds and proteins. Trade names include Santophen 1, Septiphene, Chlorophen and Ketolin.

chlorophyll
This green chemical is what makes it possible for plants to photosynthesize (turn light into food). It's used in cosmetics for its antiseptic, antifungal and odor-absorbing qualities, and also in very small amounts as a natural color.

chlorothymol
This *phenolic compound,* a chlorine derivative of *thymol,* is used in mouthwashes as an antiseptic. Thymol on its own isn't irritating to most people, but when combined with chlorine, it's very irritating to the mucous membranes and can also cause skin rashes. You should avoid it.

chloroxylenol
This preservative, used in deodorant soaps, hair conditioners and children's cosmetics at concentrations between 0.5% and 2%, has been found to be a primary skin irritant. It's a halogenated *phenolic compound* synthesized by treating 3,5-dimethylphenol CL2 with xylenol. Its trade name is Ottasept. It's listed in *The British Pharmacopoeia* (1976), and registered with the EPA and the FDA.

cholagogue
In herbology, a substance that increases the flow of bile into the intestines.

cholesterol
This *steroid alcohol* is used as an *emulsifier* and lubricant in hairdressings, shampoos, conditioners and other cosmetics. It's not toxic when used topically, though it can be greasy to hair and skin if used in large amounts. Plant cholesterols are obtained from cocoa beans and myrrh, animal cholesterol from sheep wool. Human *sebum* (skin oil) is high in cholesterol and cholesterol *esters* (4.1%).

chromosome
Found in the nuclei of all cells, these rod- or thread-like bodies contain *genes.*

chrysarobin *(goa)*
This tree *(Andira araroba),* which grows in Bahia, Brazil, has yellowish wooden canals in which a powder is deposited as the tree ages. The powder is scraped out (no need to cut the tree down), mixed with splinters and other debris, sifted, ground, dried, boiled and filtered. The result is called goa powder.

Added at a ratio of one gram to an ounce of carrying agent (it should never be used full-strength), goa is a classic herbal treatment for *acne,* oily skin, *eczema, psoriasis* and other skin diseases. It's also used in moisturizers for oily skin, and mixing 2% goa into a natural ointment makes a treatment for hemorrhoids.

Even after purification, goa powder is irritating, and should be used in small concentrations. It also permanently stains clothing (although a formula exists for treating acne and oily skin that won't stain). Also see *araroba* in the herb chart in Chapter 2.

cinnamal
This derivative of cinnamon bark oil is used in cosmetics as an *aromatic* and flavoring. See *cinnamon* in the herb chart in Chapter 2.

citric acid
Derived by fermentation of crude sugars from citrus fruits, citric acid is used as a flavoring agent in foods and pharmaceuticals, and as a preservative, acid, sequestrant, foam-stabilizer and *pH*-adjuster in cosmetics. It's nontoxic.

clay
Various clays are used in face masks and especially recommended for oily skin because of their drawing properties. Deep-cleansing and highly absorbent, clay can be drying if used too frequently. *Kaolin* and *bentonite* are the two clays most commonly used.

cloflucarban
This toxic carbanilide compound (trade name: Irgasan CF3) is used as a preservative and disinfectant in cosmetics. In aerosols, its concentration is usually 0.2%; in deodorants and soaps, 1.5%.

cnidium *(Cnidium officinale)*
In China, the rhizome of this plant (known as chuanchiung) is used as a sedative and *analgesic*, and in herbal skin formulas. See *ching-shang*.

coagulant
A substance that increases clotting of the blood. Opposite of *anticoagulant*.

coal tar
A thick liquid or semisolid byproduct of the distillation of bituminous coal. Though claimed by some to have healing properties, coal tar is allergenic, *phototoxic* and harmful to the environment. Also see *certified colors* and *colors*.

cobalt chloride
This *FD&C coal tar* color is probably a carcinogen. Also see *colors*.

cocamide DEA, MEA and MIPA
Synthetic *nonionic surfactants*. See *alkyloamides*.

cocamidopropyl betaine
This synthetic *amphoteric surfactant* is frequently referred to as natural and "from coconuts" on the labels of shampoos. It's a secondary *surfactant,* used in combination with other, stronger surfactants. Also see *sodium lauryl sulfate*.

coceth-6-8
This synthetic chemical, composed of polyethelene *glycols* of coconut alcohol, is used as a cleanser and *emollient* in shampoos. It can cause allergic reactions and is harmful to the environment.

cochineal
This natural red dye is obtained from the dried bodies of the female cochineal beetle *(Dactylopius coccus),* which is native to Central and South America. Also see *carmine*.

cocoa
This familiar brown powder is made from the roasted kernels of ripe seeds of *Theobroma cacao* (and other

species). It's used for its chocolate flavor. Some people are allergic to it.

cocoa butter

This solid fat, which is expressed from the seeds of the cocoa plant *(Theobroma cacao)*, is used in lipsticks, eyelash creams, rouge, soaps and *emollient* creams as a lubricant and skin softener. Some people are allergic to it.

coco-betaine

This synthetic *amphoteric surfactant* is frequently referred to as natural and "from coconuts" on the labels of shampoos in health food stores.

coconut fatty alcohol and coconut fatty acids

These natural chemicals, obtained from *coconut oil,* are used in creams, soaps, shampoos and other cosmetics.

coconut oil

This white, semisolid fat, expressed from the kernels of coconuts, is used as an *emollient* and to make natural soaps (through a saponification reaction with salts). Various synthetic chemicals are often added to coconut oil to create cosmetic ingredients like cocoampho-carboxymethylhydroxypropylsulfonate. Our advice is: if it's too long to read, then it's synthetic and doesn't belong on your hair and skin.

cocotrimonium chloride

This *quaternary ammonium* compound is used as an antiseptic and preservative. Also see *quaternary ammonium salts.*

cocoylsarcosinamide DEA

A synthetic "coconut" derivative used as a *surfactant.* Also see *alkyloamides.*

cod liver oil
This pale yellow fatty oil is obtained from the fresh livers of the codfish (family *Gadidae)*, especially the species *Gadus morrhua.* It's extremely high in vitamins A and D, but its odor limits its use in cosmetics.

coix *(Coix lachrma-jobi)*
The seeds of this herb, known in China as i-yi-jen, are used for their cooling effect on the skin, as a *diuretic* and antirheumatic, and as an ingredient in products that treat skin pigmentation problems. See *ching-shang* and *tang-kuei.*

cold cream
Cold cream was developed by the Greek physician Galen around 150 A.D. in Rome, and was one of the early commercial cosmetics. His formula called for 55.5% almond oil, 24.5% *beeswax,* 14.5% water and 5% *rosewater.* Galen's slaves worked around the clock creating small batches, because the cream, though in great demand, was unstable.

Cosmetic manufacturers who came after Galen discovered that by adding about 0.5% *borax,* a whiter and more stable cream could be made. Later on, various synthetic chemicals and petrochemicals like petrolatum, *Tween* 40, *mineral oil,* glyceryl monostearate and *ozokerite* were added to Galen's original formula.

cold waving of hair
This method of waving the hair doesn't use externally applied heat. It began in 1930 with the "overnight cold wave process." Ten years later, a fast cold wave process based on *bisulfates* was introduced, but this was quickly replaced with a lotion that contains *thioglycolate.*

These chemicals affect the *keratin* in the hair in an adverse way, leading to serious hair damage and, in some cases, baldness. See the entry on *permanent waves* in this chapter and the natural hair-care methods described in Chapter 4.

collagen

One-third (70%) of the body's connective tissue in the *dermis* is made of collagen, and gerontologists have found that this is where the aging process of the skin takes place. There are two types of collagen, soluble and insoluble. Young connective tissue is made up of soluble collagen whose molecules are displaced in relation to each other.

As the skin ages, and is exposed to sunlight, chemicals (like makeup, *coal tar* dyes, etc.) and various foods, the soluble collagen becomes "cross-linked," so the molecules are no longer displaced in relation to each other. Cross-linking makes the collagen insoluable and inflexible. As this happens, the connective tissue slowly loses its ability to absorb moisture and becomes tight, dry, wrinkled and aged.

colloidal sulfur

This pale yellow, dried mixture of *sulfur* and *gum arabic* is a natural ingredient used for hair and scalp problems like dandruff and *psoriasis,* and to treat acne.

cologne

A kind of *toilet water* made of *alcohol* and aromatic oils, cologne may be natural or synthetic.

colors

Coloring a cosmetic is often a marketing and packaging decision that has nothing to do with the function of the product on your hair or skin; it's just a way to hopefully get more customers to buy the cosmetic by making it appear more attractive. This unnecessary coloring is of no value whatsoever; it's harmful to our health as well as to the environment (since coloring agents harm the earth and water).

A list of colors whose safety isn't known (or even studied) was made in 1960 by the *FDA* (the federal Food and Drug Administration). Although this "provisional list" was supposed to be abolished, to date nothing has been done and the colors are still being used. Ralph Nader has been questioning the safety of colors for several years and has listed most of them as unsafe.

Almost all *FD&C* (food, drug and cosmetic) and *D&C* (drug and cosmetic) colors are made from *coal tar,* which has been shown to cause cancer in animal tests. In addition, many people are allergic to coal tar. *Aniline,* a coal tar derivative, is a poison.

Because children became ill from the colors used in candy and popcorn, the FDA removed from its *GRAS* (generally recognized as safe) list FD&C Orange #1, Orange #2, Red #32 (in 1950) and, more recently, Red #1 and Yellow #1, #2, #3 and #4. In 1973, Violet #1 was removed. In 1976, the most widely used FD&C color, Red #2, was removed because it caused the growth of tumors in lab rats, and Red #4, which was used to color candy and maraschino cherries, was banned as carcinogenic. (Also see *certified colors* and *hair coloring.)*

Many people avoid any food, drug or cosmetic that contains FD&C and D&C colors, because they know them to be toxic. I agree, especially since there are many natural alternatives: annatto, *beet powder, beta carotene, caramel, cochineal,* grapeskin, *henna* and so on. Certification of these natural colors isn't needed, since they require less processing and have a long history of use.

One example of a nontoxic, natural color that rarely causes skin irritations is the oldest known dye—indigo. It's made from the indigofera plant, which is found in Bangladesh, Java and Guatemala. Indigo FD&C Blue #6 is an example of this color.

Here are some D&C and FD&C colors that should particularly be avoided for the sake of your health and that of our environment:

Azo dyes, also known as monoazo dyes, are made from diazonium compounds and *phenol*. Although they're toxic and are absorbed through the skin, they're widely used in cosmetics. If you become sensitized to hair dyes containing a chemical known as paraphenylene diamine, you'll be extremely allergic to azo dyes as well.

The *anthraquinone* family of coal tar dyes, which includes *Ext. D&C* Violet #2, is made from phthalic anhydride and *benzene*. This nightmare chemical mixture prevents the growth of cells, and causes tumors in lab rats, as well as serious skin rashes.

Only a few of the toxic *nitro dyes* have been certified, because they can be absorbed through the skin. When this happens (or when they're ingested), they can cause a lack of oxygen in the blood, and liver damage. What's more, they're harmful to the environment.

Quinoline, which is derived from coal tar, is highly toxic and carcinogenic. It contains *formaldehyde,* acetaldehyde and aniline—all poisons (and I bet you thought if you didn't see formaldehyde on the label, you didn't have to worry about this toxic chemical. D&C Yellow #10 and #11, and many other artificial colors, are made with quinoline.

Triphenylmethane dyes (sometimes called tritan) are used to color many cosmetic products. They're made from carbon tetrachloride, benzene and aluminum chloride—which are highly toxic and carcinogenic. Some examples are FD&C Green #1, #2 and 3#, and FD&C Blue #1.

Xanthenes are a group of bright colors used for lipsticks; they include FD&C Red #3, D&C Red #2 and #19 (also called Rhodamine B) and D&C Orange. *Xanthenes* are toxic and cause *phototoxicity* of the skin (which can lead to skin cancer).

compound
A substance formed by the chemical union of two or more elements.

concentration
How much of something is in something else (usually expressed as a percentage or as *ppm)*.

concretes
Wax-like substances prepared from bark, flowers, roots, herbs and leaves, concretes are primarily used in perfumery and in the preparation of *absolutes*.

contact dermatitis
Skin damage caused by topical contact with chemicals.

copal
This natural *resin,* obtained from tropical trees of the species *Leguminosae* or dug up as fossils, is used in cosmetics as a thickener.

copolymer
See *polymers*.

coptis *(Coptis chinensis)*
Known in China as huang-lien, the root of this plant is used as a digestive aid, and in herbal mixtures to treat skin problems. See *ching-shang*.

corn acid
This mixture of *fatty acids* derived from corn oil is used in cosmetics as an *emollient* and thickener.

corn oil
This yellow, semidrying, fatty oil is obtained from the wet milling of corn. It's used in soft soap and as an *emollient* and thickener in cosmetics.

cortisone
This powerful *steroid hormone* is produced in our bodies by the adrenal cortex, and is synthesized industrially for the treatment of disease. Prolonged use of cortisone can lead to calcium loss in the bones, destruction of *collagen* and a weakened immune system.

cosmocul CG
This *cationic* preservative and disinfectant is used in cosmetics at concentrations of 0.2% to 1.0% of a 20% solution. It's toxic and a primary skin irritant. (In lab tests, rainbow trout were murdered with 10 ppm, and rats showed retardation of growth after ninety days on 6.2 ppm.) It's sold under the trade names Cosmocil 20% solution and Vantocil IB.

cottonseed oil
This pale-yellow, semidrying, fatty oil is obtained from the seeds of the cotton plant by solvent extraction or expression. Cottonseed oil is high in glycerides of *linoleic, oleic* and *palmitic acids* and is used as an *emollient* in cosmetics.

counterirritant
In herbology, a substance that causes an irritation in order to counteract an irritation elsewhere in the body.

couperose
This word is used by *aestheticians* to describe a condition of the skin in which capillaries are broken.

cross bonds
Cross bonds hold together the long chains of *amino acids* that compose the hair. These chains can be broken down by external environmental conditions, over-processing or the use of harsh, synthetic hair care products.

C12 C18 alcohols
These long-carbon-chain *fatty alcohols* can be natural or synthetic; examples are cetyl, palmityl, myristyl, stearyl, arachidyl and oleyl. They act as moisturizers and carrying agents for skin and hair products. Also see *cetyl alcohol*.

cutaneous
Pertaining to or affecting the skin, particularly the *dermis* (which is also called the *cutis)*.

cuticle
The outermost layer of the skin; also called the *epidermis*. Also refers to the fold of skin at the base of the fingernail.

cutis
Another name for the *dermis*.

cysteine
This sulfur-containing *amino acid* is present in the hair protein *keratin,* where it forms the "cysteine bond"

(sometimes also called the "cysteine bridge"). When hair is permed, colored, toned, bleached, straightened, braided or chemicalized, the vital cysteine bond is quite often destroyed, thereby causing hair damage—and sometimes hair loss.

Topical application of cysteine may help strengthen and repair damaged hair, so look for it in shampoos and hair conditioners. (In addition to its beneficial effect on hair, cysteine is said to stimulate the immune system.)

Also look on your shampoo and conditioner label for two herbs that are high in cysteine—*horsetail (Equisetum aruense)* and *coltsfoot (Tussilago farfara)*. Both contain silica as well as cysteine. See the section on natural hair care in Chapter 4.

damar gum
This gum, which is extracted from an East Indian pine of the genus *Agathis,* is used largely in printing inks and varnishes. Also see *gums.*

D&C
When this abbreviation precedes the name of a color, it means that the *FDA* has certified it as safe for use in drugs and cosmetics, but not in food. (The term *Ext. D&C* means the color can only be used externally, and not around the eyes or inside the mouth.)

D&C colors are usually synthetic, *coal tar* colors; they're toxic and should be avoided. Compare *FD&C,* and see *colors* and *certified colors.*

dandruff
Clumps of cells which form on the scalp and flake off are called dandruff. Although the exact reasons for it aren't known, a good natural shampoo, conditioner

and hot oil treatment can help. See the section on natural hair care in Chapter 4.

Dantoin 685

This preservative is a *nonionic* compound containing *formaldehyde* (19%) and N-acetal. Used in shampoos (at concentrations of 0.2%) and in deodorants, it's highly toxic, as are all formaldehyde solutions. Since the formaldehyde is split off at a *pH* of 6 in water solutions, Dantoin 685 actually amounts to free formaldehyde.

Dantoin 685 is stable at low temperatures. It's supplied as crystals that are soluble in water and alcohol. The cosmetics industry can list it on labels as DMDM hydantoin, but this doesn't tell consumers who want to avoid formaldehyde that *this is formaldehyde*. See *formaldehyde*.

DEA *(diethanolamine)*

This liquid amino alcohol, which is similar to *TEA* (triethanolamine), is used to alcoholize cosmetics. You should avoid it, since it may be contaminated with *nitrosamines*. See *nitrosamines* and *alkyl sulfates*.

DEA-lauryl sulfate

This synthetic *anionic surfactant* is used extensively in shampoos. It does *not* come from coconuts, and may be contaminated with *nitrosamines*. Also see *alkyloamides*.

DEA-linoleate

This *salt* of *linoleic acid* plus *DEA* is used as a cleanser. It may be contaminated with *nitrosamines*. Also see *alkyloamides*.

decoction
A diluted aqueous extract prepared by boiling a *botanical* with water for a specific period of time, then straining or filtering it.

decyl alcohol
This colorless or light yellow liquid is a primary *alcohol* that may be natural (made from coconut oil) or synthetic. It's used in *surfactants* and perfumes as an *emulsifier* and *emollient*.

dehydroacetic acid
This synthetic crystalline *acid,* used as a *fungicide, bactericide* and *plasticizer,* is toxic.

demulcent
In herbology, a substance that soothes irritated tissues, particularly mucous membranes.

deodorant
In cosmetics, a product that reduces perspiration odor. There are natural deodorants containing herbs like marigold and *vitamin E.* Note that deodorants don't stop perspiration; that's the role of an antiperspirant.

depilatories
Although hair is a strong fiber, these extremely *alkaline* cosmetics destroy it by breaking the chemical bonds that hold it together. After using any hair removal method, a moisturizer should be applied to soothe the skin.

depressant
A substance that reduces nervous activity.

depurative
In herbology, a detoxification substance that purifies the blood or an organ.

derivative
A particular substance or group of substances that is removed from a "donor" substance.

dermabrasion
In this process, skin is removed (in varying amounts and depths) by means of mechanical brushes or sandpaper. It's used to remove scars and as a final treatment for *acne hypertrophica*.

dermatitis
Inflammation of the skin caused by an allergic reaction, dermatitis is often caused by coming in contact with a cosmetic product that has numerous synthetic ingredients. Certain people may be allergic to natural substances as well.

dermatologist
One who understands and has been trained to treat diseases of the skin, especially with drugs.

dermis
A sensitive layer of skin, protected by the *epidermis*, that's made up of connective tissue, muscle and nerves. It's also called the "corium" or "true skin."

desiccant
A drying substance. Also called an *exsiccant*.

detergent
These synthetic soaps may be made with a variety of chemicals, and are frequently not biodegradable. Known in the trade as *syndets* (synthetic detergents)

and *surfactants,* they're harmful to the environment. Also see *alkyloamides.*

diammonium citrate
This synthetic chemical, used as a preservative, sequestrant and *astringent* in cosmetics, should be avoided.

diaphoretic
In herbology, a substance that produces perspiration.

dibromopropamidine
This benzamidine compound is a toxic chemical. Lab mice were murdered with intravenous doses of 10 mg/kg and with subcutaneous injections of 300 mg/kg. Its trade name is Brolene.

dibutyl phthalate
This colorless, oily *ester,* used as a *plasticizer* and solvent in cosmetics, is a synthetic chemical that should be avoided.

di-calcium phosphate dihydrate
An *abrasive* commonly used in toothpaste.

dichloro-M-xylenol
This toxic *phenolic compound* is used as a substitute for phenol in baby cosmetics and soaps, at concentrations of 0.1%.

dichlorophene
Like other *phenolic compounds,* dichlorophene can accumulate in the *stratum corneum* and is potentially neurotoxic. The European Economic Community suggests cosmetic concentrations of 0.2% in soaps (with a maximum concentration of 1%). When used in a cosmetic, the label must warn: *contains dichlorophene.* Its trade names are DCP, G-4 and Preventol GD.

diet for hair & skin

Obviously, what you eat has plenty to do with how you look, as well as how you feel. The choice of a sensible diet can do wonders for your skin, giving it a healthy glow and texture that no cosmetic can. Conversely, dull-looking skin and dry, lackluster hair are often due to a bad diet, an excess of chemicalized foods, or synthetic chemicals in cosmetics.

A diet heavy in starches and sugar is acid-forming in the body; this contributes to premature aging of the body. Salt is one of the worst chemicals you can use in your diet. The skin already contains a large amount of salt, which is eliminated in perspiration. Salt in your diet only increases this problem and causes wrinkles and dry skin. It should be avoided.

To keep your cells hydrated, you should drink about six glasses of water a day. Drink pure water or distilled water, not tap water. You can also get your water in an herb tea or vegetable broth.

Fresh vegetables and fruits, whole grains, beans and herbal teas are the best sources of vitamins and minerals. A lack of vitamins A and C, the B vitamin riboflavin and trace minerals leads to rough, scaly, wrinkled skin and a muddy, pasty complexion. Proteins are also important, as are the *essential fatty acids,* both of which retard the appearance of wrinkles.

Vitamin A keeps hair and skin soft and supple, and the nails strong. Spinach and carrots are rich in it.

Vitamin C is needed to help the blood carry oxygen to the skin cells, and aids in the formation of *collagen.* A deficiency of it leads to an older appearance. Take at least one gram(1,000 mg) a day.

Riboflavin helps prevent large pores. When it's insufficient, young people are susceptible to blackheads and older people to wrinkles around the mouth.

The sulfur-containing *amino acids* are important to hair and skin. You can get them from protein-rich foods, and from Brussels sprouts, lentils and onions.

I believe every cosmetic should contain some amount of vitamins A, C and E. Even if only a small amount is absorbed into the skin and utilized by the skin cells and the blood, continual use will improve the skin and hair from the inside out, as well as from the outside.

diethanolamine
More commonly known by its abbreviation, *DEA,* diethanolamine is one of many synthetic detergents. Like *TEA* (triethanolamine), it may be contaminated with nitrosamines and should be avoided. See *nitrosamines* and *alkyloamides.*

diethylene glycol
This synthetic *glycerin* is used as a *humectant,* solvent and *surfactant.* Kidney, liver and central nervous system damage can result from oral doses of less than one ounce of this toxic chemical.

diethyl phthalate
This colorless, odorless *ester* is used as a solvent in perfumes, a *plasticizer* in nail polishes, as an insect repellent and as a *fixative.* This synthetic chemical can irritate the mucous membranes, and absorption through the skin can cause depression of the central nervous system, leading to unconsciousness and coma.

digestive
In herbology, a substance that helps digestion.

dihydroxyacetone

This synthetic chemical, which contains *acetone,* is used in quick-tanning products to dye the skin brownish-orange. What it does when it's absorbed into the body is unknown. Since it alters skin, it should have a drug status, and its *FDA* approval should be questioned.

diisocetyl adipate

This synthetic compound of hexadecyl alcohol and adipic acid is used as buffer.

dilauryl thiopropionate

This synthetic compound of lauryl alcohol and 3,3'-thiopropionic acid is used as *antioxidant.* Also see *propionic acid.*

dimethicone

This silicone fluid is used to give a smooth feel to a cosmetic cream or lotion. Silicones were very popular during the 1960's, but various allergic reactions and internal problems make them questionable as cosmetic ingredients. Although they're still widely used, they should be avoided. Many herbal oils, such as vegetable glycerine, can easily replace this chemical.

dimethoxane

This dioxin compound is used to preserve cutting oils, *resin* emulsions, water-based paints and as a gasoline additive; in cosmetics, it's used at concentrations of 0.1%. Dioxin products are toxic and a danger to the environment. Its trade name is Dioxin CO.

dimethyloldimethylhydantoin

This toxic compound, which contains 17.7% *formaldehyde,* is used as a preservative in detergents, shampoos, cream conditioners and hand creams in concentrations from 0.15%, and against yeast and molds at concentrations of 0.4%. (As with most formaldehyde products, it has a broad spectrum of activity against bacteria, but higher concentrations are needed against fungi.)

It can be listed on labels as DMDM hydantoin, but this doesn't tell consumers who want to avoid formaldehyde that this is a formaldehyde product.

A *nonionic* liquid with a formaldehyde odor, it's soluble in water and is compatible with *anionics, cationics,* nonionics and proteins. Its trade names are Dantoin 55% solution, DMDMH-55 and Glydant. It's often combined with *parabens* and *inorganic salts* like 5-chloro-2-methyl4-iso-thiazoline-3-on and 2-methyl-4-iso- thiazoline-3-one (Kathon CG). See *formaldehyde.*

diphenolic acid
This aromatic *alcohol* is used as a *surfactant* and intermediate in cosmetics. It's a synthetic *phenolic compound* that's irritating to skin, eyes and mucous membranes, and it should be avoided.

diphenylene sulfide
This toxic *phenolic compound* is used as an antiseptic.

disinfectants
Disinfectants free the surfaces on which they're used from infection; they usually destroy vegetative matter and harmful organisms. *Essentials oils* (like lavender oil) sometimes have disinfectant properties. See the herb chart in Chapter 2.

disodium monococ-laureth
This synthetic *fatty acid alcohol* (plus *sodium)* is used as a *dispersant* and a *surfactant,* usually in shampoos. It

can cause allergic reactions, is harmful to the environment and should be avoided. Also see *fatty alcohols*.

dispersant
An agent that helps one substance disperse into another, and/or that helps stabilize such a dispersion.

diuretic
A substance that increases urination.

DMAE
See *PABA*.

DMDM hydantoin
See *Dantoin 685* and *dimethyloldimethylhydantoin*.

dolomite
This naturally occurring mineral is used as an abrasive in cosmetics. It consists of calcium magnesium carbonate, but it can be contaminated with other substances and heavy metals, so it should be avoided.

domiphen bromide
This quaternary ammonium salt is used as an antiseptic and as a preservative.

Draize test
This test, devised in 1959 by J. H. Draize, is used extensively by the chemical and cosmetic industry to test the eye-irritancy of chemicals. The chemical to be tested is dripped into one eye of a rabbit but not the other (which serves as a control).

The rabbit is held in a device that prevents it from shaking its head or scratching the eye that's been doused with the chemical. Albino rabbits are used because their tear ducts are less efficient than those of other rabbits at washing the irritating chemical away.

The Draize test is used to torture many millions of animals every year; the statistics derived from their suffering end up on technical data sheets that are used to sell chemicals to companies that manufacture cosmetics and other products.

drug

According to the Federal Food, Drug and Cosmetic Act (as amended), the term *drug* means:

a. articles recognized in the official United States Pharmacopoeia, the official Homeopathic Pharmacopoeia of the United States, the official National Formulary, or any supplement to any of them

b. articles intended for use in the diagnosis, cure, mitigation, treatment or prevention of disease in human beings or other animals

c. articles (other than food) intended to affect the structure or any function of the body of human beings or other animals

Cosmetic manufacturers aren't allowed to use any labeling (including product brochures, which are also considered labeling) that suggests that their products are drugs—that is, that they're therapeutic, will cure disease, or will alter a body function.

dryness of skin and hair

Dry skin is flaky, dull-looking and feels too tight; dry hair is lusterless, fly-away and straw-like. Dryness of the skin or hair can be caused by insufficient *essential fatty acids* in the diet, or by hair- and skin-care products that strip away natural oils or inhibit the body's ability to re-oil itself after washing or shampooing.

It's best to use a moisturizer on your skin and a conditioner on your hair, regardless of the soap, cleanser or shampoo you use. For more details, see Chapter 4.

eczema
This acute or chronic inflammation of the skin is characterized by red, scaling, itching and oozing lesions; it's usually non-contagious. Most treatments for *eczema—steroid* creams, for example—are synthetic and irritating to the skin. One natural treatment found to help eczema is *evening primrose oil,* taken internally and applied externally.

edema
Abnormal accumulation of clear, watery fluid in the lymph spaces of the connective tissue.

EDTA
This is an acronym for *ethylene diamine tetra acetic acid,* a synthetic chemical that's used as an an *antioxidant* and as a "complexing" agent in shampoos—which means that it binds metallic ions so that the *surfactants* can work more effectively. Similar compounds are disodium EDTA and trisodium EDTA. All are toxic and should be avoided.

EFAs
An abbreviation for *essential fatty acids.*

effleurage
A light, stroking movement used in massage.

8-hydroxyquinoline
This toxic, *coal tar* chemical is used (in the form of potassium hydroxyquinoline sulfate) as a topical antiseptic in skin creams and lotions, in concentrations between 0.05% and 0.5%. It's *phototoxic* and may cause cancer (some coal tar colors have been found to be carcinogenic in animal tests). It must bear a warning on the label that reads: *Not for sun protection*

products, and it isn't allowed at all in products for children under three years old.

Quinoline is obtained by the oxidation of *aniline* and *glycerine* (the same process used to make artificial colors). It's supplied as a yellow (sulfate) or white (sulfate-free) crystalline powder. Trade Names are Bioquin, Chinosol and Quinosol. Also see *colors.*

elastin

This dermal protein, similar to *collagen* and *reticulin,* is used as an *emollient* in some natural cosmetic formulas. It's typically an animal byproduct (usually bovine), but there are herbal (vegetarian) alternatives.

elixir

This term describes a clear hydroalcoholic liquid used orally in homeopathic medicine(sweeteners are often added).

emetic

A substance that causes vomiting and is usually used to detoxify.

emmenagogue

A substance that promotes menstrual flow.

emollients

These substances, used *topically,* prevent water loss, and thus have a softening and soothing effect on the skin. They can be natural, like almond oil, or synthetic, like *mineral oil.*

emulsifiers

Also known as *emulsifying agents,* these substances promote the formation of, and stabilize, *emulsions.* Emulsifiers can be natural or synthetic.

emulsion

A homogeneous mixture in which small globules of one liquid are suspended in another liquid with which it won't mix. Salad dressings, for example, are emulsions of oil in vinegar or lemon juice.

endocrine glands

These organs secrete *hormones* directly into our bloodstreams. Examples are the thyroid, adrenals and pituitary.

epidermis

The outer, protective layer of the skin, which covers the *dermis*. Also called the *cuticle*.

EPO

An abbreviation for *evening primrose oil*.

essential amino acids

Amino acids that can't be manufactured by the body.

essential fatty acids

Sometimes known as *vitamin F* (and often abbreviated *EFAs)*, these substances can't be manufactured by the body and must be consumed in the diet. There are three types—linoleic, linolenic and arachidonic.

The essential fatty acids fulfill many functions in our bodies. They lubricate, aid in the transportation of oxygen to the cells, help coagulate the blood, combine with *vitamin D* to make calcium available to the tissues, regulate glandular activity, break up *cholesterol* deposits on arterial walls, maintain healthy mucous membranes and nerves, assist in the assimilation of phosphorus and help convert *carotenoids* to *vitamin A*.

The more saturated fats we consume, the more important it is to increase our intake of EFAs. The National Research Council recommends at least 1% of the daily caloric intake, and this figure should probably be higher. Excellent sources for unsaturated fatty acids are raw wheat germ, raw sunflower seeds, butter and cold-pressed vegetable oils.

Essential fatty acids are used in the production of *sebum,* your skin's own natural oil, so including these substances in skin care products makes good sense. The essential fatty acids tend to be *bacteriostatic.*

essential oils
The odor-bearing constituents of plants, essential oils are complex mixtures of *alcohols, ketones, phenols, acids,* ethers, aldehydes, *esters,* oxides and *sulfur* compounds (among others). They're also called volatile oils, ethereal oils, essences or *absolutes.*

ester
An *organic* compound formed from an *acid* and an *alcohol,* an ester is the organic equivalent of a *salt.*

esthetician
See *aesthetician.*

estrogen
This female sex hormone is usually synthesized for drug use. The use of hormones externally or internally is dangerous. Also see *hormone.*

ethanol *(or ethyl alcohol)*
This colorless, volatile liquid with a burning taste is well-known to most of us as the active ingredient in alcoholic beverages; in fact, ethanol is commonly

called simply "alcohol," although there are many other kinds of alcohols.

Ethanol is widely used in cosmetics as a solvent and as an antibacterial agent. As a preservative, it's effective at concentrations of 15% to 20%. It's a disinfectant in concentrations of 60% to 70%, with a bactericidal effect within 45 seconds. It's also used in acne treatments and in rinses for oily hair.

Ethanol absorbs water and thus can be very drying to the skin, hair and scalp. It's used in *astringents* and in fast-drying skin lotions (at concentrations of 15%); the lotions need to include *glycerols* and vegetable oils to reduce the drying effect.

A 50% alcohol solution provokes a delayed allergic reaction in some people when used *topically.* Taken orally, ethanol is toxic in doses above 80g.

Ethanol is often deliberately made poisonous by the addition of *methanol* and it is then known as SDA (specially denatured alcohol). Its sale is regulated by the Alcohol and Tobacco Tax Department of the federal government. Specially denatured alcohol is given numbers based on the amount of denaturants used (i.e. SDA 40).

Ethanol is *miscible* with water, *acetone* and *glycerol.* It's produced by the fermentation of sugar or starch or by the hydration of ethylene, which is an acrylate *copolymer.* (Acrylics are very toxic synthetic plastic *resins.*) It's difficult to know by reading a label whether an alcohol is natural or synthetic.

ethoxydiglycol
This toxic solvent, used in nail polishes and lacquer thinner, can be a skin irritant.

ethoxyethanol
This is a synthetic *alcohol* plus ethoxy, which is a hydrocarbon and a byproduct of the natural gas industry. It's used as a solvent. Absorption can cause kidney damage and depress the central nervous system.

ethyl acetate
This synthetic *ester* of *ethyl alcohol* and *acetic acid* may irritate the skin and depress the central nervous system. It's used as a solvent in many industrial products, and is found in nail polishes and nail polish removers.

ethyl alcohol
See *ethanol*.

ethyl paraben
See *parabens*.

eucalyptol
This thick, syrupy liquid is the chief component of eucalyptus oil; it's also found in Levant wormseed and cajeput. Also known as cineole, it's used for its antiseptic, flavoring and aromatic qualities. See the herb chart in Chapter 2.

eugenol
This colorless, *aromatic*, liquid *phenol* is found in many *essential oils*, especially cinnamon-leaf and clove oils. It's used as a flavoring, in perfumes and as a disinfectant and pain reliever in dentistry.

European Economic Community
Also known as the Common Market (and commonly abbreviated EEC), this union of European countries works to reduce tariff barriers and promote trade between its members. The EEC sets standards for cos-

metic ingredients and labelling that are often different from those in the US.

evening primrose oil

This *essential oil*, often referred to by the abbreviation *EPO*, comes from the yellow evening primrose, *Oenothera biennis* (it's called the *evening* primrose because its flowers only open at night). EPO is available in health food stores as a liquid, as a cream, in capsules and as an ingredient in cosmetics. It's been extolled by herbalists as a treatment for:

- alcoholism
- arthritis
- brittle nails
- diaper rash (evening primrose cream works best)
- eczema (I've found it quite effective when EPO is applied first as an oil, and an evening primrose cream is put on top of that; for infants, just use the cream)
- hyperactivity in children (according to the Feingold Institute, even the small amount absorbed by using the cream topically is very helpful)
- multiple sclerosis
- premenstrual syndrome (I've been told by many women that it works)
- psoriasis (I've found it helpful in breaking up the large, crusty lesions)
- schizophrenia

In early 1981, a rumor circulated that EPO helped weight loss, and people began flocking into health food stores to buy it. Did it work? I don't know, but I got a call from one woman who said she lost 25 pounds when she took the oil for eczema (EPO can be used internally as well as externally for eczema).

EPO is high in *essential fatty acids,* especially a rare one called *gamma-linolenic acid (GLA).* GLA is usually formed in the body as part of the process of creating hormonelike substances called prostaglandins (also known as *PGs).*

Because there are so many prostaglandins, it's not known exactly what they all do. One that has been fairly well documented is PGE1, which has been shown to lower blood pressure, open up the blood vessels, relieve the pain of angina and prevent thrombosis. (Dr. Ulf von Euler of Sweden and Dr. M.W. Goldblatt, working independently, discovered the effect of PGs and their ability to reduce blood pressure as early as 1930.)

When prostaglandins are concentrated in certain areas of the brain, they stimulate the release of substances known as neurotransmitters, chemicals that are used by the brain and nervous system to transmit all its messages. So EPO functions as a "smart drug" (as does any other nutrient that stimulates the production of PGs).

To create prostaglandins, you need GLA. To produce GLA, certain essential fatty acids must be present in the foods you eat. If you're consuming the wrong types of fat in your diet, the process of manufacturing GLA—and thus PGs—is interrupted. Saturated fats, for example, will destroy essential fatty acids. Other inhibitors to the production of GLA are a high consumption of alcohol and deficiencies of *pyridoxine* (vitamin B6), niacin (vitamin B3), *ascorbic acid* (vitamin C) and the mineral *zinc.*

It's also possible to ingest GLA directly. Some researchers have said that EPO is the only dietary source for GLA, but in fact it can also be found in borage oil (where its concentration is higher than 10%) and in black currant seed oil.

The *topical* use of EPO seems to improve the skin (as do many essential fatty acids). As mentioned above, it's best to first apply the oil and then apply the cream over it. (The oil shouldn't be used near the eyes.) In shampoos and hair conditioning sprays, EPO removes tangles and repairs damaged hair, and it adds a natural, nongreasy luster as well.

EPO is highly acidic and can burn the soft tissues of the mouth, so when taking it orally, always mix it with juice or water. The usual dose is fifteen drops. Also see the herb chart in Chapter 2.

expectorant
A substance that promotes the release of mucus from the lungs and the air passages.

expression
Pressing or squeezing out, as an oil from a seed.

exsiccant
A drying substance. More commonly called a *desiccant*.

Ext. D&C
When this abbreviation precedes the name of a color, it means that the *FDA* has certified it as safe for use only in drugs and cosmetics, not in food, and only externally, not around the eyes or inside the mouth.

Ext. D&C colors are usually synthetic, *coal tar* colors; they're toxic and should be avoided. Compare *D&C* and *FD&C,* and see *colors* and *certified colors.*

extracts
Extracts are generally, but not necessarily, concentrated forms of natural substances obtained by treating

raw materials with a solvent and then removing the solvent completely or partially from the preparations. Extracts may be solid, powdered or *tinctures.* Also see *native extracts,* and the herb chart in Chapter 2.

F.
Abbreviation for Fahrenheit, the temperature scale (used pretty much only in the U.S.) in which water freezes at 32° and boils at 212°. Compare *C.*

facials
Facials (treatments of the skin of the face) are usually done in beauty salons with a whole variety of synthetic products. It's impossible to know the ingredients, because they don't have to be listed for salon products. You can give yourself a natural facial at home with natural products; for a step-by-step explanation of how to do that, see the section on natural skin care in Chapter 4.

fats
Fats are a class of chemical compounds that are insoluble in water but are soluble in *alcohol,* ether, the glycerides of one or more *fatty acids,* and other solvents. Obtained from rendered animal fat, oil seeds or fruit pulp, they're used as *emollients* in cosmetics. Fats can be solid, semisolid or liquid.

fatty acid esters
These *esters* of *unsaturated fatty acids* yield *resins* that are used in many industries. In cosmetics, they're often used to compound synthetic fragrances or as flavors. There's the possibility of allergic reactions to some chemicals used in the esterification process (a condensation reaction in which the molecule of an acid unites with a molecule of alcohol, with the elimi-

nation of a molecule of water). The alkyl salt of carboxylic acid is an example of a fatty acid ester.

fatty acids
Saturated aliphatic monocarboxylic acids is the chemical term for these *organic* oils that are found in vegetable and animal fats. They can be either *saturated* (e.g. *palmitic, stearic)* or *unsaturated* (e.g. *oleic, linoleic,* linolenic).

Fatty acids frequently occur in the form of *esters* and glycerides and are obtained by hydrolysis of fats or by synthesis. They're excellent *emollients* for the skin and an important part of the diet (especially in the form of *essential fatty acids).*

fatty alcohols
These *alcohols* of cetyl, lauryl, oleyl and stearyl *fatty acids* are thick to semi-thick, syrup-like liquids with high *emolliency.* They can be natural or synthetic, and are sometimes used in hair and skin conditioners, creams, lotions and conditioning shampoos.

favus
This parasitic fungus disease that attacks the scalp of humans is characterized by yellowish, dry incrustations resembling a honeycomb. Regular use of an herbal hair rinse and conditioner containing the herbs *horsetail* and *coltsfoot* can be helpful.

FDA
The Food and Drug Administration, the federal agency responsible for regulating the safety and efficacy of all foods and drugs sold in the US.

FD&C

When this abbreviation precedes the name of a color, it means that the *FDA* has certified it as safe for use in food, drugs and cosmetics. Compare *D&C* and *Ext. D&C*, and see *colors* and *certified colors*.

febrifuge

In herbology, a substance that reduces or stops a fever.

fermentation

The chemical decomposition of *organic* compounds into a simpler compound through the action of enzymes or certain bacteria.

ferric chloride

Made by boiling iron in chlorine, ferric chloride is used in medicine and cosmetics as an *astringent* or *styptic*. It's available as a *tincture* or in a water solution, and it may irritate the skin.

ferric ferrocyanide

This dark-blue powder, also known as Prussian blue or iron blue, is exceedingly toxic.

ferrous sulfate

This *astringent salt* of iron is used in cosmetics as an antiseptic and in medicine to treat anemia. It's a suspected carcinogen.

fingernails, care of

Fingernails are composed of *keratin* (a protein also found in hair). The hard nail plate isn't living tissue, but the bed it rests on contains blood vessels. The fold of skin at the base of the nail is called the *cuticle*.

The fingernails have traditionally been decorated in various ways. Long, decorated fingernails are a sign of wealth and leisure, since they're difficult to maintain in jobs that require manual labor. Because the nail is so tough, nail polishes, nail polish removers and cuticle removers are among the most caustic and damaging of cosmetics. There are practically no natural nail products.

Application of rose hip oil, white camellia oil and *evening primrose oil* can strengthen nails, and the intake of cysteine, an amino acid, can improve fingernails. Also see *amino acids, cysteine, rose hip oil* and *white camellia oil.*

5-bromo-5-nitro-1,3-dioxane (Bronidox L)

This extremely toxic preservative is so corrosive that it will eat right through metal containers. It's an active ingredient in propylene glycol and in a compound known as o-Acetal, o-formal. The European Economic Community suggests using it in cosmetics at concentations of 0.1%.

fixatives

Fixatives are materials that retard the evaporation of the more *volatile* components in perfume formulations. They're usually of a high molecular weight, and have a high boiling point.

fixed (fatty) oils

These are chemically the same as *fats,* but they differ physically in that they're generally liquids at room temperature.

fluoride

Flourides are compounds of the element fluorine. Although toxic, they're used in toothpastes as an anti-enzyme ingredient to retard tooth decay, and are added to the water supply in some states and localities.

follicle
A small cavity or depression in the skin that contains the hair root.

formaldehyde
A suspected carcinogen, this colorless, pungent, irritating substance is found in many preservatives, such as the hydantoins; it's also used as a disinfectant. It's acutely toxic when inhaled or swallowed, and 44% of all people whose skin is exposed to it get a toxic reaction.

At one point, the FDA banned formaldehyde from cosmetics, but it's now used in shampoos at concentrations of 0.1% to 0.2%. If its concentration is greater than 0.05%, the European Economic Community requires that formaldehyde be identified on a product's label, but this isn't required in the U.S.

Methanol is sometimes added to formaldehyde at a 15% concentration to prevent *polymerization*.

Formalin
A trade name for *formaldehyde*.

formic acid
This toxic *organic acid* is a colorless liquid with a pungent odor. Avoid all contact of formic acid with the skin. A 10 g dose is dangerous, and a 50–60 g dose is lethal. The European Economic Community limits its concentration in cosmetics to 0.5%.

Formic acid has been used as a food preservative since 1865 in the form of sodium, potassium or calcium formate, but this isn't allowed in the United States. Formic acid has a *pH* of 3.5. It was first observed by Fischer in 1670, in ants.

Formol
A trade name for *formaldehyde*.

forsythia *(Forsythia suspensa)*
In China, this fruit is known as lien-chiao. It's used as an *anti-inflammatory* and to treat skin problems. See *ching-shang*.

4-isopropyl-3-methylphenol
Since this is a *phenolic* substance, it should be regarded as toxic. Manufactured in Osaka, Japan, it goes under the trade name of Biosol.

freckle
A yellow or brown spot on the skin, usually caused by sunlight.

fruit acids
As their name suggests, these acids are found in various fruits and herbs. Also known as *alpha hydroxy acids*, red fruit acids and amidroxy fruit acids, they're used in masks and moisturizers for their ability to exfoliate and moisturize the skin.

The principal *fruit acids* are *citric, glycolic*, malic and *lactic*. Usually associated with milk, lactic acid is also found in some plants—milk thistle, *shea butter* and coconuts, for example. The other fruit acids are mainly found in citrus fruits, apples, bilberry, black currant and sugar cane.

Fruit acids are used in concentrations as low as 0.25% and as high as 8%. The higher concentrations increase the "heat" of the product and the peeling action, but can also cause skin irritation in some people.

fuller's earth
This kind of clay is used for its moisturizing ability. It can often be found as an ingredient in facial mud pack treatments.

fungicide
A substance that kills fungus.

g
The abbreviation for a *gram*.

gamma-linolenic-acid
A *fatty acid* found in evening primrose oil, black currant seeds, borage oil and mother's milk. Also see *evening primrose oil*.

gardenia (Gardenia florida)
This fruit is known in China as chih-tzu. It's an *anti-inflammatory* and is used for skin problems in herbal formulas. See *ching-shang*.

gel
A colloidal suspension of solid and liquid particles that exists in a solid or semisolid state.

gelatin
Purified protein from animal sources used as a thickener and film-forming agent.

genes
The unit of a *chromosome* which transfers an inherited characteristic from parent to offspring.

Germall II and Germall 115
When used in concentrations of 0.5%, these toxic antibacterials inhibit and sometimes kill both gram-negative and gram-positive bacteria. The antimicrobial activity of Germall II is better than Germal 115.

Neither of the Germall products have a good anti-fungal activity and must be combined with PHB *esters (parabens)*. In cosmetics, they're used at concentrations of 0.1% to 0.5%, in combination with parabens.

These chemicals caused acute oral toxicity to lab rats at 5.2 mg/kg, and to mice at 7.2 mg/kg. Rabbits had severe *edema* and erythemas (redness and irritation) on abraded skin. Mice had fetotoxic reactions at 300 mg/kg. Germall II is diazolidinyl *urea* and Germall 115 is imidazolidinyl urea. These chemicals are compatible with *anionics, nonionics* and proteins. Germall 115 releases *formaldehyde* at over 10°C. Other trade names are Biopure 100 and Euxyl K 200.

germicide
A germ-killing substance.

g/kg
Grams per *kilogram.*

GLA
Abbreviation for *gamma-linolenic acid.* See *evening primrose oil.*

glucose glutamate
This *ester* of glucose and glutamic acid (an *amino acid)* is used as an *humectant.*

glutaraldehyde
This dialdehyde compound is an oily liquid stabilized with *ethanol* or hydroquinone. Used in cosmetics at concentrations of 0.02% to 0.2% (of a 50% solution), it's a toxic chemical that causes *contact dermatitis* in humans. The lethal dose in lab rats is 60 mg/kg. Its trade names are Alhydex and Ucarcide.

glycereth
This polyethylene *glycol* ether of glycerine is a synthetic form of *glycerine.*

glycerin, glycerine or glycerol

All three names refer to a sweet, syrupy *alcohol* that can be produced synthetically from propylene alcohol or naturally derived from vegetable oils. Glycerin has been used in cosmetics for thousands of years as a solvent, *plasticizer, humectant, emollient* and lubricant.

glyceryl coconate, dilaurate, erucate, hydroxystearate, monostearate, myristate, oleate, ricinoleate, sesquioleate, stearate, trimyristate, etc.

These *esters* of *fatty acids* combined with *glycerine* are generally used in the same ways that glycerine is. They're largely synthetic chemicals with perhaps a drop or two of some natural fatty acid in them.

Glyceryl oleate is used as an *emulsifier;* glyceryl stearate SE acts as a texturizer in pasta products and as an *opacifying agent* in shampoos, creams and lotions. They can cause allergic reactions and should be avoided.

glyceryl monoglyceride

This distilled *fatty acid* (90% monoglyceride) is a good-grade antimicrobial agent that's approved as an *emulsifier* in foods by the *FDA.* It's also used as a base lotion for pharmaceuticals and at concentrations of 0.5% in deodorants, soaps, powders, medicated shampoos, hand and foot care products, dental and gum care products. It causes some allergic reactions.

The fatty acid content gives this chemical a waxy, paste-like appearance. It's soluble in water after melting at 86° C. Compatible with most emulsifiers, it's inactivated by sodium lauryl sarcosine and some *nonionics.* It's active against gram-positive bacteria, but not against gram-negative bacteria (the harmful sort)—except when combined with *EDTA, lactic acid, parabens,* etc. Its trade name is Lauricidin.

glycine
This *amino acid* may be produced naturally (from the hydrolysis of proteins) or synthetically (from the reaction of chloroacetic acid and *ammonia*). It's used as a texturizer.

glycogen
Because this animal starch can be quickly converted to protein, it's the principal form in which carbohydrates are stored in animal tissues. Glycogen (often obtained from oyster shells) is used in hair care products to help damaged hair.

glycol stearate
This *ester* of *glycol* and *stearic acid* is used as an *opacifying agent,* thickener and pearlizing substance in shampoos, lotions and detergents (both cream and liquid). It contains up to 4% ethylene glycol and can't be considered natural. It can cause allergic reaction and should be avoided.

glycolic
A semi-thick to light oil extract of a plant. See *essential oils* and *glycosides*.

glycolic acid
This *organic acid* occurs in unripe grapes and sugar beets, but it's usually manufactured from chloroacetic acid. Glycolic acid is used as a skin care treatment in exfoliation creams and masks, and as an acidifier. Because it may irritate mucous membranes and cause allergic reactions, it should be avoided.

glycols

Glycerine is combined with *alcohols* to form these syrupy *humectants*. They can be vegetable or animal, natural or synthetic. When used in makeup, they help the foundation adhere to the skin.

Some glycols, like diethylene glycol and carbitol, are dangerous; they're absorbed into the skin and can cause allergic reactions. Ethylene glycol has caused bladder stones and is a suspected carcinogen in bladder cancer. Propylene glycol is considered safe by the *FDA* and is used widely to formulate cough syrups and other drugs, but it's still a petrochemical and should be avoided.

Avoid products whose labels don't make it clear that they're using vegetable glycerine and simply say *glycol* without the source listed. Also see *The fine art of reading a label* in Chapter 3.

glycosides

Widely present in plants, glycosides are a very important group of natural products and constitute an important source of drugs like digitalis, sennosides, ginseng and rutin. In cosmetics, they're used as moisturizing agents for the hair and skin. (See the herb chart in Chapter 2.)

Glycosides contain sugar and, when hydrolyzed, yield one or more sugars. They contain two components: glycone and aglycone. Glycone is the sugar compound (e.g. glucose, arabinose, xylose) and aglycone is the nonsugar compound (e.g. *sterols,* tannins, *carotenoids,* quinones).

glycyrrhizic acid

An *organic acid* derived from licorice root. See *licorice* in the herb chart in Chapter 2.

goa
See *chrysarobin.*

gram
A unit of weight in the metric system. There are about 28 grams to the ounce.

grapefruit seed oil
The extracted oil of grapefruit seeds is a safe natural preservative used in cosmetics. It works in both oil and water products, and has been combined with various herbal and vitamin extracts .

One processor of this extract (Dr. Jacob Harich of Chemie Research and Manufacturing) claims that it reduces bacterial infections in livestock when used as a feed additive, thus eliminating the need for antibiotics. He also claims good results using it to treat herpes (though his research into this use has been confined to South America).

GRAS list
A list, compiled by the *FDA,* of ingredients that are "generally recognized as safe" for use in foods, drugs and/or cosmetics.

green soap
This soap, made from linseed oil and the hydroxides of sodium and potassium, is used in the treatment of skin diseases, especially acne. It's often found in a soft state or as a *tincture.*

green tea
The leaf of the *white camellia (Camellia sinensis)* is used to brew the common tea we drink. If the leaves are fully fermented before being dried, the resul t is called black tea, far-and-away the most common type

in the U.S. and Europe. If the leaves aren't fermented before being dried (or are only slightly fermented), the result is called green tea; it's widely used in Japan, China and India.

Green tea has recently been discovered to have many nutritional and healthful qualities—for example, it contains 20 times the *antioxidant* effect of vitamin E. When used in facial creams and lotions, green tea increases the effect of sunscreens, and it's been found to prevent skin cancer from UV rays as well.

A special green tea is used in some cosmetics for this purpose. Called *matcha,* it's high in methylxanthines, which are believed (by the National Cancer Institute) to prevent skin cancer. Matcha can be traced back to the Sung dynasty in China, over two thousand years ago.

Green tea also helps prevent irritation of the skin caused by *glycolic acid* and other irritating chemicals that are used in skin peels and facial masks. Green tea even has anti-cellulite properties.

guaiazulene
Another name for *azulene.*

guanine
This natural pearlizing agent is made from fish scales or ground-up pearls.

gums (acacia, arabic, benzoin, guar, damar, karaya, locust bean, rosin and tragacanth)
Gums are polysaccharides of high molecular weight that are dispersed in water (i.e., they're hydrocolloids). They're superior to synthetic *polymers* like the

PVP/PVA copolymers. Some of the gums used as hair sets and natural thickeners are *acacia, tragacanth, quince seed* and *locust bean.*

gum resins
Also known as oleogums, gum resins (such as myrrh gums, gamboge and asafetida) are used in some natural cosmetics.

hair bulb
The lower extremity of the hair.

hair coloring
Both natural and synthetic dyes are used in hair coloring products, and many contain toxic chemicals. Also see *colors.*

hair follicle
The depression or cavity in the skin that contains the root of the hair.

hair papilla
A small cone-shaped elevation at the bottom of the *hair follicle.*

hair pilus
The hair itself.

hair root
The part of the hair within the *hair follicle.* Compare *hair shaft.*

hair shaft
The segment of the hair that extends or projects beyond the skin. Compare *hair root.*

hair texture
The density, general quality and feel of the hair, described with such terms as fine, medium, coarse, dry, normal and oily.

hamamelis water
A distillation of *witch hazel,* with added water and *alcohol (Hamamelis virginiana* is the Latin name for witch hazel).

hectorite
This mineral is one of the principal constituents of *bentonite.*

helix
The rim of skin and cartilage that goes around most of the external ear.

hematite
This naturally-occurring, color-imparting mineral, used in ancient times as a makeup powder, is again finding favor as a natural makeup product.

hemostatic
A substance that halts bleeding.

henna
This ancient type of hair coloring is made from the henna herb *(Lawsonia alba),* whose red-orange leaves contain 1% of a coloring agent called lawsone. Henna is mixed with *indigo* and logwood to obtain various shades; adding *walnut extract* and coffee creates a dark, brownish red that's quite attractive.

Adding enough *citric acid* to obtain a *pH* of 5.5 will make the color last on the hair longer. See the herb chart in Chapter 2.

hepatic
An agent that works on the liver.

herb
A plant without woody tissue that withers and dies (to the root) after flowering—particularly one used in medicine, cosmetics or foods. See the herb chart in Chapter 2.

hexachlorophene
This highly toxic chemical is used as an antibacterial agent in soaps, cosmetics and deodorants. Hexachlorophene was linked to infant deaths and brain damage in the late 1960s and early 1970s and must now carry a label warning that reads: *Not to be used on babies.*

Acutely toxic by mouth, hexachlorophene is harmful to nerves and accumulates in the *stratum corneum* (the outermost layer of the skin). pHisohex, a *topical* disinfectant cleanser that contained hexachlorophene, is no longer on the market due to toxic reactions.

Hexachlorophene is a *phenolic compound,* and is supplied as a white, free-flowing powder that's essentially odorless. Some trade names for products that contain it are Gamophen, G-ll and Hexosan.

hexahydrotriazine
People who are sensitive to *formaldehyde* can have a severe reaction to this toxic chemical. *Contact dermatitis* often occurs, as well as other allergic reactions. The European Economic Community limits its concentration in cosmetics to 0.3%. Concentrations of 69.5 ml/l killed rainbow trout within 96 hours.

Hexahydrotriazine is sold under the following trade names: Bacillat 35, Bakzid 80, Grotan BK and KM 200. The full chemical name of this n-acetal compound is tris-hydroxyethylhexahydro-triazine.

hexamethylenetetramine
This toxic chemical is a *formaldehyde* n-acetal compound that causes sarcomas when injected into lab animals. When present in a product, the label should include the wording: *Warning: Contains formaldehyde.* Trade names include Aminoform, Cystamin, Formid and Uritone.

hexamidine isethionate
This toxic benzamidine compound is used in cosmetics at concentrations of 0.1%. It's also used as a *topical* antiseptic. Trade names include Desomedine, Esomedina, Hexmedine and Hexamidin.

hexanol
Also known as hexyl alcohol, this chemical, found in the seeds and fruits of *Heracleum sphondylium* and *Umbelliferae,* is used in antiseptics and perfumes.

hexetidine
This toxic, n-acetal compound is widely used in mouthwashes (at concentrations of one gram per liter)for its local anesthetic, antibacterial and oral disinfectant effects. In pharmaceuticals, 100 mg of hexetidine in 100 ml of solution is used against *Candida albicans* (yeast) infections. Trade Names are Hexatidine, Hexetidine and Hextril.

hexyl alcohol
See *hexanol.*

hexylresorcinol
This toxic, *phenolic astringent,* derived from petroleum, causes allergic reactions.

hives
A condition in which there is an eruption of itching on the skin. Hives are often allergic.

hoelen *(Poria cocos)*
This fungus, known in China as fu-ling, is used in herbal medicine as a *diuretic* and *sedative,* and also for skin pigmentation problems.

homosalate or homomenthyl salicylate
This synthetic chemical is used to replace the *phenolic compounds* used in sunscreens. Poisoning has been reported when it's absorbed into the skin.

hormone
Hormones are secretions of *endocrine glands* that are distributed in the blood stream or in bodily fluids to stimulate specific effects in other parts of the body. Although hormones are often used as drugs and in topical treatments, they can alter the function of the body's own hormones and may cause cancer. Avoid them.

humectant
A substance, like *glycerol* or *sorbitol,* that's used to retain moisture. Using a natural humectant in a cosmetic product helps speed moisturization to the skin.

hydrate
As a noun, this means a compound formed by the union of water with another substance. As a verb, it means to supply water to something that absorbs it.

Hydrating the skin is an important step in a facial treatment (typically the face is steamed or sprayed with water, vitamins, herbs and minerals).

hydrocarbon

A chemical compound that contains only carbon and hydrogen atoms. This large group includes *paraffins,* olefins, acetylenes and alicyclic and aromatic hydrocarbons; petroleum, natural gas and coal products are all hydrocarbons.

Many synthetic cosmetic ingredients are hydrocarbon derivatives (such as *mineral oil,* propylene *glycol, coal tar colors,* etc.). Hydrocarbons from petroleum (and its byproducts) are potentially allergenic and *phototoxic,* and they harm the environment. Hydrocarbons also occur naturally in *essential oils.* Also see *colors.*

hydrochloric acid

Also known as muriatic acid, this corrosive chemical is present in gastric juice (in dilute form) and is used in cosmetics as an *oxidant* and solvent. It's also used in nail bleach. Inhaling its fumes can irritate mucous membranes.

hydrocortisone

This *hormone,* produced in the adrenal gland, is synthesized for medical use, particularly for application to inflamed skin. It can adversely affect the skin by damaging the *collagen* of the connective tissues.

hydrogenated oils

Although hydrogenating oils (adding hydrogen to them so that they're solid at room temperatures) allows them to be stored for long periods without refrigeration, it also destroys *essential fatty acids* and fat-soluble vitamins.

hydrogen peroxide
This explosive, corrosive compound, used in cosmetics as an oxidant, bleach and antiseptic, is a primary irritant and can cause blisters on the skin.

hydrolyzed animal protein
This ingredient is included in many shampoos for its ability to improve hair, repair split ends and impart luster to the hair. Careless manufacturing can contaminate the protein.

hydrophilic
Having the ability to unite with or attract water. A hydrophilic cosmetic ingredient (panthenol, for example) will attract moisture to the skin.

hydroquinone
This *phenolic compound,* derived from *benzene,* is used in skin bleaches, and also as an *antioxidant* and *antiseptic.* It's a potential skin allergen, and ingestion of even tiny amounts can result in nausea and vomiting. Ingestion of less than one ounce can be fatal.

hydrotheraphy
The scientific treatment of disease through the use of water. Also see *balneotherapy.*

hydroxyamine HCL
This synthetic compound, which is used as an *antioxidant,* contains *hydrochloric acid;* it can be severely allergenic and a skin irritant.

hydroxyethylcellulose
This synthetic *polymer* is used as an *emulsifier* and *plasticizer*. Also see *cellulose gum*.

hydroxyproline
This nonessential *amino acid* is found in large quantities in *collagen,* and it's believed to be helpful to the skin's collagen when applied *topically.*

hygroscopic
Capable of absorbing moisture from the atmosphere; readily absorbing and retaining moisture.

hyperidrosis
A state of excessive sweating.

hypersensitivity
Abnormal reactions to drugs or other external substances.

hyponychium
The portion of the *epidermis* upon which the fingernail or toenail rests.

indigo dye
See *colors*.

indole
This crystalline compound, found in jasmine oil and civet, is a product of the decomposition of proteins containing the *amino acid tryptophan*. Although indole has an unpleasant odor, it's used as a trace ingredient in perfumes.

ingest
To take into the body by mouth.

inflammation
A reaction of the body to irritation, marked by redness, itching, swelling, heat and pain. Skin problems of this type can be allergic reactions to *topical* cosmetics.

ingrown hair
A hair that grows underneath the skin. Ingrown hairs can cause infections.

ingrown nail
The growth of the nail inward towards the skin instead of outward towards the finger or toe. It can cause pain and possibly an infection.

inorganic
Matter not related to, and lacking the structure of, living organisms. In chemistry, inorganic pertains to compounds that don't contain *hydrocarbons* but do contain oxides and sulfides of carbon. Compare *organic.*

inositol
This B vitamin, usually associated with choline, occurs naturally in *lecithin* (which the body produces). As part of lecithin, inositol helps metabolize fats and dissolves *cholesterol.* Although more inositol is found in the body than any other nutrient except niacin, no minimum daily requirement for this substance in human nutrition has been established. Also see *vitamin B complex.*

insoluble
Incapable of dissolving or very difficult to dissolve. Also, in reference to *collagen,* incapable of absorbing moisture.

in vitro
This term refers to experiments carried out in an artificial environment, outside of living organisms. (Literally, it means "in glass"—in other words, in a test tube, laboratory flask or similar type of equipment.) Compare *in vivo*.

in vivo
Within a living organism, as opposed to *in vitro*. Here's an example of how these two terms are used: "Sure, it worked *in vitro*, but that doesn't necessarily mean it will work *in vivo*."

iodine
This nonmetallic element occurs in seawater and in plants and animals that grow in the sea. Iodine is necessary for correct functioning of the thyroid gland; when applied *topically*, it has antiseptic benefits.

ion
An atom or a group of atoms that carries an electrical charge. Positive ions are called cations and negative ions are called anions.

ionization
By utilizing an electric current, an *aesthetician* can force positive *ions* through a moisturizing cream or lotion to assure deep penetration into the skin during a facial treatment.

Irgasan DP 300
This chemical, which is used in shampoos, soaps and deodorants, is *phototoxic,* environmentally toxic (because hydrocarbons pollute the air, water and land), and may be carcinogenic (because it's a *coal tar* derivative). Another name for this diphenyl ether compound (also known as a biphenyl) is *triclosan.*

iron oxides

Also known as jewelers' rouge, or simply as rust, these compounds are used as colorings in some cosmetics. Also see *colors* and *hematite*.

isopropyl alcohol

This synthetic *fatty alcohol,* made from propylene and sulfuric acid, is used as an antiseptic, a solvent, a rubbing alcohol and as a source for *acetone*. Also see *alcohol*.

isopropyl lanolate, laurate, linoleate, oleate, palmitate, stearate and isostearate

These *esters* of *isopropyl alcohol* and various *fatty acids* are synthetic chemicals that can irritate and cause allergic reactions.

isopropyl myristate

This synthetic chemical is used as an *emollient* and a lubricant, and to reduce the greasy feel caused by the high oil content of other ingredients. It can cause allergic reactions and should be avoided. See *fatty alcohols*.

jaborandi

A *tincture* extracted from the leaves of this South American tree (genus *Pilocarpus)* stimulates the *sebaceous gland* of the scalp. It can also be used to stimulate sweating, and was once used in hair tonics and skin hydrating products. Although poisonous if taken internally, it has no known toxicity on the skin.

Japan wax

See *waxes*.

jasmine absolute

This *absolute* is often called the "natural perfume," because it's usually obtained without *volatile* solvents or heat. Some people are allergic to jasmine.

jojoba butter *and* oil

Obtained from the jojoba shrub *(Simondsia chinensis),* which grows in the southwestern United States, this butter can be used in cosmetics as an *emollient* and in sun care products (it protects against UV rays).

Mexican and American Indians have been using jojoba oil, a liquid wax pressed from the jojoba bean, for hair and skin care for many years. See the herb chart in Chapter 2.

jojoba wax

See *waxes*.

juglone

This is the active coloring principle in walnuts and is used in hair dyes. It's not known to be toxic to the skin, but it's a poison if taken internally.

kangaroo paw flower

This spring-flowering herb, related to the amaryllis, is used in Australia in hair sprays. It's not known to be toxic.

kaolin

Because this fine mineral *clay* remains white after firing, it's used in manufacturing high-grade porcelain, paper, paint, cloth, soaps and many powdered and covering cosmetics. It's also used for its dehydrating and *astringent* effect. It's also known as China clay.

kelp
This giant Pacific marine plant, *Macrocystis pyriferae,* is high in many nutrients. It's used in some cosmetics as an *astringent.*

keratin
This insoluble albumoid (fiber protein) can be found in horny tissues like the hair and nails. High in sulfur, it's quite strong, but it is subject to chemical penetration.

keratoma
A callus, wart or any horny growth.

keratosis
A disease of the *epidermis* indicated by the presence of growths of the horny layer of tissue.

ketones
These *aromatic* substances, used in nail polish removers, are toxic. They're derived by the *oxidation* of secondary alcohols. Also see *acetone.*

kg
The abbreviation for *kilogram.*

kilogram
A measure of weight in the metric system, equal to a thousand *grams,* or about 2.2 pounds.

kohl
In ancient Egypt, this black powder was made from the ash of frankincense; later, it was made from powdered antimony (a metallic element). In the Middle East and India, kohl has been used to darken the eyelids for over a thousand years. When made from frankincense, kohl isn't known to be toxic, but minerals such as antimony can be contaminated with arsenic, phosphates and other impurities. Also see *mascara.*

Kummerfeld's lotion

This natural lotion (named after its formulator) was created in 1940 for the treatment of acne. It contains camphor, *gum Arabic, glycerine,* sulfur and rosewater.

To make Kummerfeld's lotion, mix two ounces of glycerine with a half ounce of camphor. Stir in an ounce of gum arabic until the lumps disappear, then add five ounces of sulfur. Stir well, and add this mixture to 21 ounces of rosewater in a clean container.

Since there are no *emulsifiers* in this formula, shake it well before using it, and keep it in the refrigerator when it's not in use. Apply it to the acne daily.

l

Abbreviation for *liter.*

labeling

The Cosmetic Labeling Act marked a major step in helping consumers become aware of what they put into their hair and rub onto their faces. Passed April 14, 1977, it requires that ingredients be listed, in descending order of concentration, on the labels of most cosmetics. Soap, however, is exempt, and flavors, fragrances and trade secrets don't have to be listed specifically. See *The fine art of reading a cosmetics label* in Chapter 3.)

lactagogue

A substance that stimulates the breasts to produce milk.

lactalbumin

Because this natural milk protein is high in *lactic acid* and contains all eight of the *essential amino acids,* it's an excellent ingredient for hair conditioners. The late Adelle Davis called it the most perfect protein.

lactic acid
This acid, which occurs naturally in milk, produces *pH* levels like those of the hair and skin; it also helps moisturize the skin naturally. See *fruit acids.*

lake colors
These solid forms of dyes are made by mixing liquid dye with an insoluble powder like aluminum oxide. They may be natural, but they're usually synthetic and are made from *coal tar.* See *colors.*

lanolin
This yellow, semisolid, fatty secretion from sheep's wool is used as an *emulsifier,* a base and an *emollient.* Although lanolin is natural and is well absorbed by the skin, there have been some reports of allergic reactions.

lanolin alcohol
This solid *fatty alcohol* of *lanolin* is used as an *emulsifier* and thickener.

lanolin oil
This is *lanolin* with the wax component removed. It's used as a moisturizer.

lanosterol
This *sterol,* derived from *alcohol,* is used as an *emollient.*

lapases
These lipolytic enzymes can hydrolyze fixed oils into *glycerine* and *fatty acid* components. *Glycolic acid* is an example.

lauramide DEA
This white, waxy, *nonionic,* synthetic chemical is used in shampoos, bubble baths and detergents as a *surfactant* and foam-builder. It may be mildly irritating to the skin, and may also be contaminated with *nitrosamines.* See *alkyloamides.*

laureth 1-40
This polyethylene *glycol* ether of *lauryl alcohol* is a synthetic *surfactant* and foaming agent.

lauric acid
This mixture of *fatty acids* was originally obtained from the European laurel, but it's now obtained from *coconut* and *palm kernel oils.* Lauric acid is used to make soaps, *esters* and *lauryl alcohol.* See *fatty alcohols.*

lauryl alcohol
This *fatty alcohol,* often derived from *coconut oil,* is used to make *anionic surfactants.* It may be natural or synthetic.

laurylmyrist-oleamidosulfo-succinate
This synthetic *fatty acid* alcohol (plus sulfosuccinic acid) is used as a *dispersant* and a *surfactant,* usually in shampoos. It can cause allergic reactions, is harmful to the environment and should be avoided. See *fatty alcohols.*

LD/50, etc.
See *lethal dose.*

lead acetate
This *inorganic salt,* made from lead monoxide and *acetic acid,* is used to dye hair (it was formerly also used as an *astringent).* It's poisonous and a carcinogen.

lecithin
This naturally occurring mixture of *stearic, palmitic* and *oleic acid* compounds is used as an *emulsifier* and *surfactant*. High in the B vitamins choline and *inositol,* it's found in egg yolk and manufactured from soy oil.

lentigo
This is a small spot of pigmentation on the skin that's unrelated to sun exposure. It may develop into a malignancy.

lethal dose
In this test, used to determine the toxicity of a chemical, batches of 100–120 animals are fed, force-fed, injected with or otherwise exposed to doses of the chemical being tested. The doses increase until half the animals are dead, which indicates that the LD/50 (lethal dose, 50%) level has been reached.

Sometimes other levels of toxicity are also determined—for example, LD/90 is the dose at which 90% of the animals die. These LD numbers are then used to sell the chemicals. Lethal dose tests are inhumane and unscientific.

leucine
One of the *essential amino acids* (i.e., it can't be manufactured by the body). Leucine is found in hair and is included in some *amino acid* shampoos.

leukoderma
This skin abnormality is characterized by a splotchy lack of pigment in bands or spots.

lime
The word *lime* on a cosmetics label can either refer to calcium oxide (often occurring with magnesia), a caus-

tic substance that's used as an *alkalizer,* or to the citrus fruit, which is used as an *astringent* or hair rinse.

limewater
See *calcium hydroxide.*

linalool
This fragrant *alcohol* occurs in many *essential oils,* especially bois de rose oil and coriander. It's used as an *aromatic.*

linoleamide DEA
This synthetic chemical (ethanolamide of *linoleic acid,* plus diethanolamine) may be contaminated with *nitrosamines.* See *alkyloamides.*

linoleic acid
This *essential fatty acid,* found in cold-pressed oils, is used as an *emulsifier* in cosmetics.

lipases
These lipolytic enzymes hydrolyze fats or *fixed oils* into their *glycerol* and *fatty acid* components.

lipids
These materials—soluble in *alcohol* (and other solvents) but not in water—include *fatty acids, fats, waxes, fixed oils,* phosphatides, cerebrosides and sometimes *steroids* and *carotenoids.* Along with proteins and carbohydrates, lipids constitute the structure of cells. When used on the skin, they have a moisturizing and *emollient* action.

lipstick
This waxy coloring that's applied to the lips may be natural or synthetic.

liter
A unit of volume in the metric system that's about 6% larger than a quart. It's abbreviated *l*.

locust bean gum
See *gums*.

loofah
This vegetable sponge is the skeleton of the loofah fruit (family *Cucurbitaceae*). Usually long and cylindrical, loofahs have a rough texture that's excellent for the body but somewhat too rough for the face.

lye
This strong *alkali*, which is made by washing wood ashes in water, is a caustic chemical that's used in drain cleaners to dissolve *organic* matter. In spite of its harshness, lye is sometimes used to make soaps. It's also used in hair straighteners, where it can burn the outer layers of the scalp and even cause blindness. Chemically, lye is *potassium hydroxide* or *sodium hydroxide*.

lysine
One of the eight *essential amino acids*.

magnesium
This lightweight mineral occurs abundantly in nature and is essential for nutrition, especially for the absorption of *calcium* and *vitamin C*.

magnesium aluminum silicate
This flaky white solid is used as an anticaking agent, filler, thickener and stabilizer in cosmetics, especially antiperspirants, creams and shaving creams. See *aluminum chemicals in cosmetics*.

magnesium oxide
Also known as magnesia, this compound is used as an *inorganic* color and *abrasive.*

magnesium silicate
Found naturally in talc, this compound is used as an anticaking agent.

magnesium stearate
This *magnesium salt* of *stearic acid* is used as a filler in cosmetics.

mannitol
This naturally sweet *alcohol,* found in plants, is used as a *humectant.*

mascara
The practice of applying black pigment to the eyebrows and eyelashes probably originated in Egypt 30 B.C. or earlier. The whiteness of the whites of the eyes was emphasized by the darkened eyelids, and the large, dark pupils appeared like black pools. The whole effect was striking.

The first black pigment used as mascara was *kohl,* originally made from the ash of frankincense, and later from powdered antimony. The Egyptians found that, in addition to adding to the natural beauty of their faces, both were soothing to the eyes.

Today, the *FDA* allows the use of pure vegetable colors, *inorganic* pigments like natural minerals and earth colors, and *lake colors* in mascara. Manufacturers must guarantee that minerals used in their cosmetics contain no more than two parts per million of any impurity such as arsenic, lead, copper, etc. *Coal tar* dyes are forbidden, even if the color is certified for use in cosmetics. See *colors.*

massage creams and oils

Massage creams and oils are popular today in *aromatherapy* massage, sports medicine and the facial and body massages given by *aestheticians*. Massage oils are usually made from a vegetable oil base. *Jojoba oil* has been used in more expensive massage oils and aromatherapy oils (as a carrying agent for the *essential oils)*, but peanut oil is the most commonly used, because it's less expensive.

Massage creams, which evolved out of the conventional *cold creams,* are usually simple in formula and often contain no *humectants*. They can be all-purpose or designed for a specific purpose. For example, a sports massage cream will probably have a heat-up and cool-down effect, which means that *menthol* and/or eucalyptus will be added to the basic formula.

Massage creams should have enough "slip" so that the hands glide smoothly over the body. At the same time, they will be absorbed (though more slowly than moisturizing creams).

matcha

See *green tea.*

MEA

See *monoethanolamine.*

melanin

This dark brown or black pigment is found in varying amounts in animals and plants. Believed to be a type of *polymer* related to *indole,* it can be derived from the *amino acids* tyrosine or l-dopa.

menstruums

Solvents, such as *alcohol, acetone* and water, that are used to extract *essential oils* from plants.

menthol

This *oleoresin,* derived from peppermint, is an excellent counterirritant and has soothing properties if used in concentrations of 1% or less.

mercury and its compounds

Mercury is a deadly poison, a heavy metal that accumulates in the body and may cause a wide variety of symptoms. Its use in dental amalgam (a silver and mercury mixture used to fill cavities) is suspected of being a health hazard, as mercury vapor is released during chewing.

Ammoniated mercury was used in bleaching cream for decades until pressure from Japan and consumer groups forced its removal. *Phenylmercuric acetate* is a highly toxic chemical used as a preservative in eye cosmetics, although it doesn't protect users from products contaminated with bacteria during use.

metallic salts

Used in men's hair restorers, these are the oldest known hair dyes. They work by coating the hair with a metallic sheath that leaves the hair dull and dry-looking. Metallic salt dyes give inconsistent and unpredictable results, and they're incompatible with permanent waves. Another toxic chemical used in some hair restorers is *lead acetate.*

Methanal

A trade name for *formaldehyde.*

methanol

A colorless, flammable, toxic *alcohol.* It's also known as *methyl alcohol* or *wood alcohol.*

methyl acetate
This *ester* of *methanol* and *acetic acid* is a synthetic chemical used as an *aromatic* and solvent. It can cause dryness and *dermatitis*.

methyl alcohol
See *methanol*.

methylcellulose
See *cellulose gum*.

methyl salicylate
This compound, which is used as a flavoring, *aromatic*, local anesthetic and *anti-inflammatory*, is the major constituent of *wintergreen oil* and sweet birch oil (at concentrations of around 98%), but it can also be produced synthetically.

mg
The abbreviation for *milligram*.

mg/kg
Milligrams per *kilogram*.

mica
This group of somewhat shiny silicate minerals that split into very thin sheets is used in eye cosmetics to provide sparkle.

microcrystalline wax
See *waxes*.

milk protein
Also known as *lactalbumin*, milk protein is derived from whey and consists largely of *casein*. It's used in natural hair conditioners. See *lactalbumin*.

milligram
A unit of weight in the metric system equal to a thousandth of a *gram.*

milliliter
A unit of volume in the metric system equal to a thousandth of a *liter.*

mineral oil
A liquid mixture of *hydrocarbons* obtained from petroleum. Allergic reactions have been reported when mineral oil is used *topically,* and it may be *phototoxic.*

mineral spirits
This flammable petroleum distillate, which is lighter than kerosene, is used as a solvent.

mineral water
Water that's drawn from a natural spring, and which may have therapeutic properties.

minimal erythermal dose
The amount of time in the sun that produces a sunburn (it varies from skin type to skin type).

mink oil
Another self-proclaimed miracle moisturizing ingredient, obtained from minks. Vegetable oils are just as good and animals aren't killed to obtain them.

MIPA
See *alkyloamides.*

miscible
Able to be mixed with.

ml
The abbreviation for *milliliter.*

ml/kg
Milliliters per *kilogram*.

ml/l
Milliliters per *liter*.

moisturizer
A substance that, when used externally on the hair or skin, raises the moisture content.

mole
A small, raised spot, mark or protuberance on the skin, usually pigmented.

molecule
The smallest unit of any substance that contains all the properties of that substance.

monoethanolamine (MEA)
This liquid amino *alcohol* is used as an *humectant* and *emulsifier* in cosmetics. It may be contaminated with *nitrosamines*. See *alkyloamides*.

monoisopropanolamides
See *alkyloamides*.

monoxide
A chemical compound that contains a single atom of oxygen in each molecule.

montan wax
See *waxes*.

montmorillonite
A clay mineral used in facial masks.

mordant
A substance—such as *alum*, *phenol* or *aniline oil*—which fixes the dye used in coloring.

morpholine
This *amine*, made from ethylene oxide and ammonia, is used as a solvent and *emulsifying* agent.

mucilaginous
Soothing to irritated or swollen skin.

mucopolysaccharide
This class of hexosamine-containing polysaccharides, widely distributed in the human body (as well as in the cells of other animals and plants), binds with water to form the thick, jelly-like material that cements cells together and lubricates joints. (The name was coined by K. Meyer in 1938, at the Cold Springs Harbor Symposium in Quantitative Biology.) The simplest molecule of mucopolysaccharide that is able to penetrate the skin is laluramina.

musk
An animal or vegetable substance used as a *fixative* in perfumes. Animal musk is obtained from a sac situated under the skin of the abdomen of the male musk deer, or from other animals like the musk-ox, civet cat and muskrat. Herbal (vegetable) musk is obtained from the musk seed *(Hibiscus abelmuschus)*, the ambrette seed *(Abelmoschus moschatus)*, the musk mallow or the musk clover. See *musk seed* in the herb chart in Chapter 2.

myristalkonium chloride
This *quaternary ammonium salt,* made from *myristic acid,* is used as a *surfactant,* antiseptic and preservative.

myristic acid
This *fatty acid*, found in nutmeg, coconut oil and sperm oil, is used in cosmetics as an *emulsifier* and foaming agent. It's also called tetradecanoic acid.

myristyl alcohol
A *fatty alcohol* derived from *myristic acid*.

myristyl lactate
This *ester* of *myristyl alcohol* and *lactic acid* is used as an *emollient*. See *fatty acid esters*.

nail polish remover
This strong synthetic chemical mix consists of a solution of *acetone* (or a related chemical) mixed with conditioning ingredients (which may include petrochemicals like propylene glycol). Acetone is a highly flammable, *volatile* solvent that can dissolve many plastics; it can be fatal if swallowed. The conditioning ingredients do little to mitigate acetone's strongly drying and degreasing effects. Also see *ketones*.

NaPCA
See *sodium PCA*.

naphthol
See *1-naphthol*.

native extracts
This term refers to botanicals extracted by a solvent (or mixture of solvents) and then concentrated under reduced pressure until all the solvent is removed. They're usually of high potency, and solid, fluid or powdered extracts of varying concentrations are derived from them.

natural
This word is even more commonly abused on cosmetics packaging than on food packaging. For a product to be natural, it shouldn't contain synthetic chemicals. To make sure, read the label (with the help of this book).

natural colors
Derived from plants (such as *indigo*) or insects (such as the *cochineal* beetle), natural colors are appropriate for use in natural cosmetics. See *colors*.

NDELA
See *nitrosamines*.

NDGA
NDGA (nordihydroguariaretic acid) is an *antioxidant* used in trace amounts in cosmetics. Whether made synthetically or derived naturally from the creosote bush, it's toxic and has caused kidney damage.

nephritic
In herbology, a substance that helps kidney problems such as nephritis.

nerol
This *aromatic alcohol* is found in a number of herbal *essential oils,* including immortelle, hops, labdanum, lemon petitgrain, lemongrass, orange and rose. Essential oils containing high concentrations of nerol, geraniol, eugenol, betapinene and/or furfurol have antimicrobial properties against *Staphylococcus aureus, Escherichia coli, Candida albicans* and a *Mycobacterium* species.

N-hexane
This toxic compound is used in concentrations of 0.01% to 0.1% in cosmetic creams, toothpaste,

deodorants and antiperspirants. To be effective at low concentrations, it's usually combined with *parabens,* chlorocresol and B-phenoxyethanol. Human studies show allergic reactions to this chemical.

Soluble in *alcohol, glycerol,* propylene *glycol,* polyethylene glycols and to some extent in water, it's supplied as a white crystalline powder. N-hexane is *cationic,* incompatible with *anionics,* various *gums,* natural soap and sodium alginate, and is unstable at temperatures above 70° C. It's sold under the trade names of Hibitane, Novalsan, Rotersept, Sterilon, Hibiscub and Arlacide.

nitric acid

This *inorganic acid* is used as an oxidizer and stabilizer in cosmetics. It's a corrosive liquid that can irritate skin; inhalation can irritate the lungs and bronchial passages. Oral doses can be fatal.

nitrites

See *carcinogenicity in cosmetics.*

nitrocellulose

This flammable synthetic substance (similar to gun cotton) is used as an *emulsifier* and protective film in cosmetics, especially nail polish.

nitro dyes

See *colors.*

nitrosamines

This class of compounds, formed from secondary *amines* by the addition of nitrous acid, have been found in animal experiments to be very carcinogenic. More than 120 N-nitroso compounds have been examined and about 80% of them have been found to be carcinogenic to some degree.

One that occurs in many cosmetics is NDELA (N-nitrosodiethanolamine). *TEA* (triethanolamine), widely used in many cosmetic formulations, is the chemical primarily suspected of creating NDELA, but all *amines* and *amides* are capable of forming N-nitroso compounds. For example, *DEA* (diethanolamine) also reacts with nitrosating agents like the ones shown in the next paragraph to form NDELA.

Here's a list of nitrosating agents that are widely used in cosmetics as dyes and perfumes:

- cocoyl sarcosine
- diethanolamine (DEA)
- formaldehyde
- hydrolyzed animal protein
- imidazolidinyl urea
- lauryl sarcosine
- monethanolamine (MEA)
- quaternium-7, 15, 31, 60, etc.
- sodium lauryl (or laureth) sulfate
- sodium methyl cocoyl taurate
- sodium nitrite
- triethanolamine (TEA)
- 2-bromo-2-nitropropane-1,3-diol

In 1978, Dr. David H. Fine (then working at the Thermo Electron Corporation in Waltham, Mass.) invented a nitrosamine-detector called the Thermal Energy Analyzer. He and his group discovered that over 40% of TEA-containing cosmetics were contaminated with nitrosamines. Little is known about the problem, but more than one consumer publication has recommended avoiding any cosmetic that contains TEA or DEA.

NDELA penetrates human skin under normal conditions of topical application. *In fact, nitrosamines in general are absorbed through the skin in far greater amounts than when nitrite-preserved food is eaten.*

To prevent nitrosamine formation in cosmetics , you can either eliminate the chemical that's capable of becoming a nitrosating agent, add an agent that prevents nitrosation reactions from occurring, or change the chemical environment—typically, the *pH*—so that the reaction between the nitrosating agent and the amine or amide won't take place.

For example, quaternary amines and amine oxides react with nitrites to form nitrosamines in an acidic medium, but not in an alkaline or neutral one. A cosmetic formula whose pH ranges between 3.4 to 4.5 and which contains nitrosating agents has the potential to develop nitrosamines. Therefore, to assure a measure of safety, low-pH and *pH-balanced* shampoos, conditioners and rinses should be free of amines and amides.

Water can be another contributing factor—sodium nitrite and 2-bromo-2-nitropropane-1,3-diol both form nitrosamines in aqueous solutions. But simply not putting sodium nitrite into a cosmetic formula may not be enough to protect the product from nitrosamines, because water in the formula can also be a source of nitrite. Ion exchangers have been suggested to remove nitrite and nitrate from water, but because the ion exchange *resins* are prepared with amines, they contain minute amounts of nitrosamines themselves.

What's more, sodium nitrite is present in the seaming compound used on the 55-gallon metal drums (both new and used) in which cosmetic ingredients are commonly shipped. Using plastic and fiberboard drums can avoid this source of contamination, but this solution isn't always practical.

The conditions under which cosmetics are prepared and the raw materials stored may also contribute to nitrosamine contamination. For example, cosmetic raw materials in half-empty drums can become contaminated with nitrogen oxides in the air.

I've used the combination of water-soluble *ascorbic acid* and fat-soluble ascorbyl palmitate (both of which are forms of vitamin C) and fat-soluble tocopherol *(vitamin E)* with great success since 1969, and have found them very effective in both aqueous and non-aqueous cosmetic formulations. (The inhibitory action of ascorbic acid and ascorbyl palmitate against nitrosamines has been well established, both *in vitro* and *in vivo.)*

Synthetic *antioxidants* such as *BHA* and *BHT* haven't yet been shown to be effective blocking agents against nitrosamines. *Phenolic compounds* are also poor blocking agents because they can combine with a nitrosating agent to form chemicals that either liberate the nitrosating agent or that catalyze nitrosamine formation itself.

References for this entry:

Archer, M.; Tannenbaum, S.; Fan, T. Y.; and Weisman, M., "Reaction of Nitrite with Ascorbate and Its Relation to Nitrosamine Formation," *Journal Natl. Cancer Inst.,* vol. 54, no. 5, 1975, pp. 1203-1205.

Dahn, H., Loewe, I. and Bunton, C. A., "Uber die Oxidation von Ascorbinsaure durch salpetrige Saa. Teil VI: Ubersicht and Diskussion der Irgebnisse," *Helv. Chim. Acta.,* Vol. 42, 1960, p. 320.

Magee, P.N., Montessano, R. and Preussmann, R., "N-Nitroso Compounds and Related Carcinogens," *C. E. Searle, Chemical Carcinogens, [ACS Monograph 173],* The American Cancer Society, 1976, pp. 491-625.

nonionic
Having a neutral electrical charge. Compare *anionic* and *cationic*.

nonoxynol compounds
This large group of ethoxylated alkyl *phenols* are widely used as *surfactants* and *dispersants*. Like all phenols, they're toxic and should be avoided.

nucleic acids
Either of two groups of complex acids (DNA or RNA) that determine the genetics of living things. These substances are added to cosmetics with the claim that they will strengthen cellular rejuvenation of the skin, but this is just a sales pitch.

occlusive agents
Occlusive agents are materials (like plastic wrap and Band-Aids) that hold strongly to the surface of the skin, increasing absorption and blocking access to the air. Occlusive agents have been used for thousands of years to speed healing of wounds and as beauty treatments.

ocotea cymbarum oil
This *essential oil,* obtained by steam distillation from the bark of a Brazilian tree *(Ocotea cymbarum),* has a high *safrole* content, and is used as a substitute for *sassafras* oil.

oils
These viscous substances, which are generally insoluble in water, are obtained from animal, plant, mineral and synthetic sources.

ointment
A semisolid preparation for the skin, usually with a fatty or greasy base.

oleic acid
This *fatty acid,* a common constituent of many animals and vegetables, is also a common cosmetic ingredient. It can be isolated from vegetable oils or produced from inedible tallow. When *hydrogenated,* oleic acid yields *stearic acid.*

oleoresins
These plant products consist of *essential oils* and *resins* in solution (examples are *gums, turpentines* and *balsams).* Oleoresins can occur naturally (Oregon balsam is an example) or they can be extracted by means of solvents from plants like paprika and ginger.

oleth-2 *through* **oleth-50**
These polyethylene *glycol* ethers of oleic *alcohol* are used as *surfactants.* They're synthetic chemicals and can cause allergic reactions.

oleyl alcohol
This *fatty alcohol,* an oily, unsaturated liquid found in fish oils or manufactured from *esters* of *oleic acid,* is used to make *surface-active* agents.

olfactory
Relating to the sense of smell.

1-naphthol *and* **2-naphthol**
These *coal tar* derivatives are used as antiseptics, parasiticides and dye intermediates. They can irritate the skin and are harmful to the environment. They're absorbed through the skin, and oral doses larger than one teaspoon can be fatal. See *colors.*

opacifying agent *or* **opacifier**
A substance that changes the appearance of cosmetics from clear to cloudy. An example is *titanium dioxide.*

O-phenylphenol
This *phenolic compound* is very toxic. Its trade names are Doxicide 1 and Preventol O.

oral
By mouth.

organic
Carbon is an essential part of every organic compound, and is necessary for all living things. In today's chemistry, the term *organic* means that the substance described contains a carbon atom. But when the term was originally defined by the Swedish chemist Berzelius, it described any substance that is, or once was, living. In this book, I follow Berzelius' definition.

origanum oil
This oil, related to marjoram, comes from the *Thymus capitatus* plant. It's used as a fragrance in cosmetics and as a flavoring in foods. It's a natural oil, but some people may be allergic to it.

orris
An *essential oil* derived from European plants of the genus *Iris,* especially *Iris pallida,* orris is used as a flavoring and fragrance. Orris root is also powdered and used in sachets, tooth powders and as a powder base.

ouricury wax
See *waxes.*

Oxadine A

This toxic *amine* substitute is used in protein shampoos and hand creams at concentrations of .05%–0.2%.

oxidation

This common chemical reaction is caused by the combination of oxygen and another substance. Fire and rust are both examples of oxidation, as is butter (or any *fat* or *oil)* turning rancid.

Oxidation is an important cause of cosmetics deterioration (as is the activity of microorganisms), though *topical* application of a product whose fats are rancid isn't as harmful as consuming one (rancid fats in the diet can destroy certain vitamins and other essential elements, and may cause cancer). *Antioxidants* inhibit oxidation, and thus protect the oil phase of cosmetics from becoming rancid.

oxyquinoline

This *aromatic alcohol,* usually derived from *coal tar,* is used as an antimicrobial. It can cause allergic reactions.

ozokerite wax

See *waxes.*

PABA

PABA *(para-aminobenzoic acid)* is a water-soluble B vitamin found in blackstrap molasses, bran, *brewer's yeast,* eggs, liver, milk, rice, organ meats, *wheat germ* and whole wheat. The *RDA* is 50–60 mg per day.

PABA is well known for its ability to screen out the burning effects of *UV rays.* Several other substances also do this job, but PABA is still the choice for sun protection. It works best when combined with other sun protectors like *jojoba butter (and oil),* African butter (also known as karite, or shea butter), *aloe vera, green tea,* willow bark extract and cuttlefish oil. Though PABA isn't easily washed away, it holds best to the skin if also combined with *fatty acid esters, sorbitol* or vegetable *glycerine.*

It's believed that PABA—combined with selenium, *vitamin C,* the *amino acid cysteine* and other B vitamins like *inositol, pantothenic acid,* folic acid, *biotin* and niacin—can retard hair loss and prevent gray hair. In any case, when used in shampoos and hair conditioners, PABA will prevent UV damage of the disulfide bond in hair (another cause of hair loss and breakage).

A *salt* of PABA known as *DMAE* (dimethyl-amino-ethanol) is an amino *alcohol* believed by some scientists to reduce the aging process by removing the accumulated toxic byproducts of metabolism. The theory is that, as we age, our bodies gradually lose the ability to create the digestive enzymes known as lysosomes, and that PABA and/or DMAE keeps the lysomal enzymes doing their job of eliminating the toxins. (However, there have recently been reports of allergic reactions to DMAE.)

The brown spots on our skin (commonly called age spots or liver spots) are a result of the accumulation of toxins within the body. When these toxins accumulate in brain cells, they interfere with cellular metabolism, which is why DMAE is said to improve mental functioning.

PABA is generally not toxic. A recent FDA regulation requires that it appear on labels as *para-aminobenzoic acid,* not simply as *PABA.*

palmamide DEA, MEA and MIPA
Combinations of *palm oil* and ethanolamides. See *alkyloamides*.

palmitate
A *salt* or *ester* of *palmitic acid* used in baby oils, bath oils, eye creams, hair conditioners and moisturizers. It causes allergic reactions in some people.

palmitic acid
Also called hexadecanoic acid, this *fatty acid* occurs in *palm oil* and most other *fats* and fatty *oils*. When used in cosmetics, palmitic acid may contain petrochemicals like propylene *glycol,* for enhanced *emulsibility.*

palm oil *(also known as* palm kernel oil*)*
This white to yellowish *fat,* obtained from palm kernels (particularly those of the African oil palm), is similar to *coconut oil* and is used to make soaps, shampoos (especially baby shampoos), ointments and margarine.

pantothenic acid
Also known as vitamin B5, panthothenic acid is found in bran, *brewer's yeast,* brown rice, carrots, cauliflower, cheese, eggs, fish, peas, legumes, lima beans, mushrooms, oats, organ meats, peanuts, *royal jelly,* salmon, soybeans, spinach, walnuts, wheat, *wheat germ,* whole grains and liver. The *RDA* is 4–7 mg, and it's not known to be toxic in any dosage.

Pantothenic acid is an excellent skin *hydrator;* used in moisturizers or complexion sprays, it leaves the skin smooth and moist. When combined with *PABA,* folic acid and *inositol,* it makes hair look thicker and fuller and gives it body; it's also said to prevent gray hair. *Gums* or *resins* are hardly needed (or not needed at all) in hair sprays that use pantothenic acid.

papain

Papain is a proteolytic enzyme (that is, a substance that breaks down proteins or *peptides* into simpler substances, as in digestion) that comes from green papayas. It's used to tenderize meat, to chill-proof beer and as a digestive aid, and it's also been used in cosmetics to soften skin.

parabens

These toxic, allergenic, synthetic chemicals are used to preserve cosmetics, but they aren't effective with shampoos or with products that contain proteins. See *PHBs*.

paraffin

This waxy, crystalline mixture of *hydrocarbons,* usually derived from petrochemicals, is used as a thickener for cosmetics. See *waxes*.

paraformaldehyde

This toxic, *polymerized* formaldehyde is sold under the trade names Formagene, Foromycen and Triformol. For toxicity data, see *formaldehyde*.

parts per million, parts per billion

One part per million means that in a million grams (ounces or whatever) of a mixture, there's one gram (ounce or whatever) of the substance being described. Parts per billion work the same way. They're abbreviated *ppm* and *ppb*.

patch test

If you're concerned about allergic reactions to a particular cosmetic, apply a small amount of it to your inner arm, cover it with a bandage and leave it for 24 hours. If redness or soreness develops, you'll know that you have an allergic reaction to some constituent of that product. If there's no redness or soreness, the product is probably safe for you to use (at least as far as allergies are concerned).

P-chloro-M-cresol
This halogenated *phenolic* antimicrobial is used as a *topical* antiseptic, a disinfectant, a preservative in pharmaceuticals, and in protein shampoos and baby cosmetics at concentrations of 0.1% to 0.2%. It's sold under the trade names of BP, PCMC and Preventol CMK. Like all phenolic products, it should be considered toxic.

peach kernel oil
This can refer to two different oils. One, which is also called *persic* oil, is obtained by *expression*. The other, a toxic *essential oil* that's very similar to bitter almond oil, is obtained by steam distillation and is used as an *emollient* or *aromatic* in cosmetics.

pectin
This natural substance, obtained from vegetables or fruits, is used in cosmetics as an *emulsifier* and thickener. It consists of partially methoxylated polygalacturonic acids.

pectoral
In herbology, a substance that provides relief from chest and lung ailments.

PEG compounds
These synthetic plant *glycols* are used as binders, solvents, *emollients*, *plasticizers*, bases, carriers, *emul-*

sifiers and *dispersants*. They cause many allergic reactions. Their name comes from the fact that they're usually polyethylene glycols, but they can also be *polymers* of ethylene oxide. See *alkyloamides*.

pentapotassium triphosphate
These *inorganic salts* are used as *emulsifiers,* sequestrants and *dispersants*. They can irritate skin and mucous membranes; they aren't biodegradable, pollute our water and are toxic to marine life.

peptides
These compounds, which can be natural or synthetic, are composed of *amino acids* linked by *peptide bonds* (the carboxyl group of one amino acid attached to the amino group of another). When *peptide* bonds in the hair are broken, damaged hair is the result.

percutaneous
Through the skin.

perfume
More concentrated than a cologne, a perfume may be natural or synthetic, but unless you know the manufacturer to be dead-set against synthetic chemicals, it probably contains them. Even high-priced French colognes and perfumes contain synthetic *essential oils* and *fixatives*. Perfumes can cause allergic reactions.

permanent waves
Cold-process permanent waves were introduced in 1941 and have been extremely popular ever since, even though the chemicals used—highly *alkaline thioglycolates*—are extremely toxic. Permanents work by using enough thioglycolates to break the protein bond in the hair without destroying the hair itself—a tricky

procedure. The hair's protein bond then reforms while the hair is rolled on curlers and the permanent wave solution is neutralized.

Not surprisingly, hair is damaged and weakened by all this, and becomes more susceptible to *UV* and chemical damage. Worse yet, the strong detergents added to permanent wave solutions to degrease the hair and allow penetration of the thioglycolates into the hair shaft also enhance absorption of this corrosive, caustic chemical into the skin.

People who get permanent waves should use a natural shampoo and conditioner daily, but that still won't be enough. Permanent waves eventually cause hair loss, and they should be avoided if you want to keep your hair.

Hair that's damaged from being "over-processed" should be treated with a hair conditioner that includes the sulfur-containing amino acid *cysteine* and/or the herbs *coltsfoot* and *horsetail*. All three help rebuild the "cysteine bond" or "cysteine bridge" which has been destroyed by the wave solution.

peroxide
See *hydrogen peroxide*.

persic oil
See *peach kernel oil*.

petroleum jelly (or petrolatum)
This familar, semisolid mixture of *hydrocarbons* is derived from petroleum. All petrochemicals pollute our water and destroy marine life. Avoiding them is essential for the health of humans, animals, fish, water, land and air.

PGs
See *evening primrose oil.*

pH
In this common measure of the *acidity* or *alkalinity* of a solution, the lower the number, the more acid the solution, and the higher the number, the more alkaline. The scale runs from 0 to 14, with 7 being neutral (neither acid nor alkaline).

pH balanced
See *acid balanced.*

PHBs *(p-hydroxybenzoic acid benzyl esters)*
These preservatives are widely used as antimicrobials in cosmetics (in shampoos, for example) under the names methyl *paraben,* propyl paraben, ethyl paraben and butyl paraben. They're incompatible with *anionics, nonionics* and proteins, and protein-containing products preserved with them have been found to contain microorganisms, even when the PHBs were used in high concentrations and the products appeared to be bacteria-free. This means that PHBs can't be safely used in any skin care product that contains *collagen, elastin, placenta, hydrolyzed animal protein, keratin,* etc.

Different PHB esters have differing amounts of antimicrobial activity, but all are acutely toxic orally. In lab tests, "higher animals" were more sensitive. It took only 3 g/kg of methyl paraben, 5 g/kg of ethyl paraben and 6 g/kb of either propyl or butyl paraben to murder dogs, while 300 g/kg was required to kill rabbits.

PHBs were first used in 1924. Supplied in the form of a white crystalline powder, they're odorless, soluble in water at 20° C and soluble in solvents. Trade names include Nipagin, Nipasol, Nipakombin, Nipabenzyl and Solbrol.

phenol and phenolic compounds
Consiting of carbolic acid and related compounds, these toxic chemicals are often used as preservatives in cosmetics.

Phenonip
This is a trade name for a blend of p-hydroxybenzoic acid *esters,* and like the *parabens* and *phenoxyetol,* it's toxic.

phenoxyetol
This *phenolic* derivative, sold under the trade names of Arosol, Dowanol EPH, Phenyl Cellosolve, Phenoxethol, Phenoxetol and Phenonip, murdered lab rats at 1.3 g/kg. Also see *parabens.*

phenylmercuric acetate
This *organic cationic,* also known as *PMA,* is a primary skin irritant. It contains mercury, a deadly poison, and when it was put in the food of lab animals, it gave them kidney disease.

PMA is used in eye cosmetics and can enter the body through the eyes or the tender skin around the eyes. Trade names for it include Advacide PMA 18, Cosan PMA, Mergal A 25, Metasol 30, Nildew AC 30, Nuodex PMA 18, Nylmerate and Troysan. Also see *mercury and its compounds.*

phloroglucinol
This synthetic color can be a severe skin irritant.

phospholipids
Any of a class of fat-soluble *organic* chemicals present in the fat deposits of all living cells (e.g. *lecithin*).

phosphoric acid
This clear, viscous liquid is used in cosmetics as an *antioxidant*, sequestrant and acidifier. It's corrosive to the skin and mucous membranes when used in a concentrated form.

phototoxic
Phototoxic substances increase the response of the skin to *ultraviolet* rays and can cause sunburn without any allergic effect being involved.

P-hydroxybenzoic acid benzyl esters
See *PHBs*.

phytocosmetic
A cosmetic made exclusively from vegetable sources.

phytodermatology
Using herbal or plant substances for the treatment of the skin, or manufacturing products from plant substances for skin care.

phytotherapy
Using plants and herbs for therapeutic purposes (either internally or externally).

piroctone olamine
Although this toxic *pyridine* derivative is compatible with many ingredients commonly used in hair care products (like *anionic, cationic* and *amphoteric* synthetic detergents), it's incompatible with many natural *essential oils*. It's used in antidandruff hair tonics

and shampoos, but there are safe, natural ingredients that will do the same job. Its trade name is Octopirox.

placenta
This organ, present in all mammals except marsupials and monotremes, unites the fetus to the mother and is expelled at birth. Bovine placenta liquid, obtained from cows between the third and fourth month of pregnancy, is used in some cosmetics as a moisturizer.

plasticizers
An agent that keeps a substance soft and/or pliable.

PMA
See *phenylmercuric acetate*.

poloxamer compounds
These two *polymers*, polyoxethylene and poly-oxypropylene, are synthetic *surfactants*. Allergic reactions to them have been reported, and they're pollutants.

polyhydric alcohol esters
These *fatty alcohol esters* are used in cosmetics as *emollients, humectants, emulsifiers* and moisturizers. They can be natural (*glycerine, sorbitol* and *mannitol* are examples) or synthetic (mono and di-fatty acid esters of ethylene *glycols, diethylene glycol,* polyethylene glycol *(PEG),* propylene glycol and polyoxyethylene sorbitol).

polymers, polymeric, polymerization
A *polymeric* compound is one in which two or more identical molecules are combined to form a complex compound with a higher molecular weight. Some polymers consist of millions of repeated, linked molecules.

Polymers are used in cosmetics to keep sunscreens from washing off, in hair-setting products, and as binders in skin creams. Plastic fingernails are also produced by polymerization. Some of the better known polymers are cellulose, acetate, *polystyrene,* polyisobutylene, polyvinyl acetone and *polyvinyl-pyrrolidone (PVP).*
Most chemical polymers can be allergens to skin and hair. PVP, for example, which is used in hair sprays and wavesets, causes dry hair and a flaking of the scalp that's similar to dandruff.

polypeptide
A *peptide* containing more than ten or so *amino acid* molecules (and sometimes as many as 100 or more).

polysorbates
These *fatty acid esters* are used in many cosmetics as *emulsifiers.* Polysorbates are assigned various numerical values—polysorbate 60, polysorbate 80, etc—according to their formulas and whether they're intended to be used in foods or cosmetics. Polysorbate 20, for example, is used as an anti-irritant in anti-sting shampoos.
Some authors have praised polysorbates for their ability to grow hair and cure dandruff, but they can be extremely drying to the scalp. If used in hair care products, they should be combined with *essential fatty acids, aloe vera* and/or other oils to offset this tendency.

polystyrene
This *polymer* of styrene may be a liquid *balsamic* oil from the bark of the Asian tree (genus *Styrax)* or a synthetic chemical. It's used in cosmetics packaging as a protective plastic film.

polyvinylpyrrolidone
This petroleum-derived chemical, commonly known as *PVP*, is used in hairsprays, wavesets and other cosmetics. Inhaled particles may cause problems in the lungs of sensitive people.

potassium
This chemical element (atomic number 19, symbol K) stands in the middle of the *alkaline* metals, below *sodium* (Na) and above rubidium (Rb) on the table of elements. At 380 parts per million, potassium is the sixth most plentiful element in sea water (exceeded by chlorine, *sodium, magnesium, sulfur* and *calcium*).

Potassium reacts even more violently to liquid acids than sodium; in fact, it verges on being explosive. Some potassium compounds are used in cosmetics (e.g. *potassium hydroxide)*, but I don't recommend putting them on your hair and/or skin.

potassium carbonate
A potassium compound used in making soft soaps. See *potassium hydroxide*.

potassium hydroxide
Also known as *lye* or caustic potash, this chemical is used in liquid soaps. In ancient times, seaweed was burned and the ash was used. Later table salt (sodium chloride) was used.

powdered extracts
These are prepared from *native extracts* by dilution to a specified strength, followed by drying, usually under vacuum. The dry solids are then ground into fine powders or into coarse granules, in combination with lactose, dextrose, sucrose or starch.

ppb
Parts per billion.

P-phenylenediamine
This solid, crystalline substance is used as an intermediate in *aniline (coal tar)* hair dyes. Highly allergenic,
it's also a potential carcinogen, and should be avoided.

ppm
Parts per million.

preen oil
The natural version of this oil is derived from ducks'
quills, but it can also be made synthetically by combining the same *fatty acids*. Preen oil has some moisturizing ability on the skin, due to ducks' ability to repel
water; in fact, preen oil is very similar to the skin's
sebum. Also see *purcellin oil*.

propamidine isethionate
This benzamidine *antibacterial*, used in *topical* cosmetics in concentrations of 0.1%, isn't stable in the
presence of *amino acids* or natural *phospholipids* such
as *lecithin*. These substances eliminate the antibacterial action and may cause adverse reactions.

propionic acid
This *organic acid*, synthesized by the fermentation of
bacteria of the genus *Propionibacterium*, is used
mainly as a preservative and antimicrobial agent in
cosmetics and food. It's a primary skin irritant, and
was used to murder lab rats at 2.6 g/kg. The trade
name is Mycoban.

prostaglandins
See *evening primrose oil*.

proteases
These proteolytic enzymes act on proteins by hydrolyzing specific *peptides*. They're used in cosmetics to soften skin and clear skin surface of cellular debris. Examples are *bromelain* (from pineapple) and *papain* (from papaya).

pseudomonas
This extremely virulent family of bacteria can contaminate cosmetic products. Preservatives are inadequate to control the problem, so care must be taken in production to make sure raw materials and finished products aren't contaminated.

psoriasis
This disease of the skin is marked by crusty patches or lesions. They can be large or small and can cover the entire body, including the scalp. Believed to be hereditary, psoriasis is the result of a rapid and abnormal growth of skin tissue. It isn't curable, but it can be controlled by the use of *UV* light, which slows down the proliferation of skin cells.

pumice
This foamy, volcanic rock is extremely light because it's full of holes. Pumice is used whole to smooth calluses, or in powdered form as an *abrasive* in cleansers. When used as a cleanser, it can scratch the skin; vegetable meals are more appropriate for this use.

purcellin oil
This is a trade name for synthetic *preen oil,* a combination of long-chain *fatty acid esters* (naturally derived or synthetically produced) that are similar to human *sebum* and to *lanolin.* Naturally-derived pur-

cellin oil is a more humane product than preen oil itself, which is taken from duck feathers.

purgative
A laxative.

PVP
See *polyvinylpyrrolidone.*

pyridine
This toxic, flammable petrochemical is used in cosmetics as a solvent. It's irritating to—and may also be absorbed through—the skin.

pyridoxine
Vitamin B6.

pyrogallic acid
This synthetic chemical is used in artificial dyes to treat skin diseases and in the chemicals used to develop photographs. It can cause allergic reactions.

quassin
This bitter crystalline principle of the Jamaican quassia plant is used in cosmetics as a denaturant, and also as an insecticide.

quaternary ammonium salts
A wide variety of these caustic *ammonium* compounds are used as water repellents, *fungicides, emulsifiers,* paper and fabric softeners, antistatic agents and corrosion inhibitors. Their use in cosmetics, especially in hair conditioners and creme rinses, came from the paper and fabric industries.

Quaternary ammonium salts may give a soft feel to the hair (and stabilize the rinse's or conditioner's emulsion), but in the long run they make hair dry and brittle. They're also allergenic and pollute the environment. A mixture of complex *lipids* such as *lecithin* and acetylcholine can be used as a natural alternative.

quaternium-15
This toxic chemical is more effective against bacteria than against molds and yeasts. One of the most used *quaternary ammonium salts,* it can cause skin rashes and other allergic reactions due to the hexammonium chloride in it. Lab rats have been murdered with doses of 0.94 to 1.5 g/kg, and mice with doses of 40 to 80 g/kg; guinea pigs had skin reactions at concentrations above 2%.

Quaternium-15 is soluble in water, *alcohol* and *glycols;* is compatible with *anionics, nonionics, cationics* and proteins; has a broad *pH* range of 4 to 10; and is unstable above 60° C. When used in cosmetic creams, it makes them yellowish in color. It goes under the trade names Dowicil 200, Dowicide Q and Preventol Dl.

quercetin
This flavonoid (don't confuse it with *quercitrin)* is present in asparagus, *catechu,* dill, elder flowers, tarragon, eucalyptus and other plants. It's the active principle of rutin, and is also known as quercetin-3-rutinoside.

quercitrin
This flavonoid (don't confuse it with *quercitin)* is present in Roman camomile, eucalyptus, euphorbias, hops, immortelle, tea and *witch hazel.* It has reportedly cured influenza *(in vitro* studies on Type A infections), increased the detoxifying activities of the liver and shown *anti-inflammatory* activity. It's also used in

cosmetics as a natural color. See *chamomile* in the herb chart in Chapter 2.

quillaya bark
The dried inner bark of a South American tree *(Quillaja saponaria)* has been used by the Indians for many years as a cleanser of the hair and as a detergent. It creates a shampoo with a soft natural lather that's good for oily scalp and dandruff. It's also known as soap bark, Panama bark and China bark. See *quillaia* in the herb charts in Chapter 2.

quince seed
The dried seeds of the *Cydonia oblonga* are used to thicken and *emulsify* cosmetics. They're also used in alcohol- or water-based hairsprays.

quinoline colors or dyes
One type of toxic *coal tar* color. See *colors.*

rancidity
This chemical decomposition of a (usually fatty) substance causes it to smell "off" or rotten. Rancidity is the result of *oxidation,* and natural *antioxidants* like *vitamins A, C* and *E* can safely slow this process.

RDA
The "recommended daily allowance"—the government's idea of how much you should ingest of a given substance.

refrigerant
In herbology, a substance that reduces excess body heat.

resins

These natural products are available either as direct plant exudates or as alcohol extractions of botanicals. They rarely occur in nature without being mixed with *gums* and/or *oleoresins*.

resorcinol

This aromatic *phenol,* used as an antiseptic, preservative and *astringent,* can be derived from *resins* such as galbanum or asafetida, but it's usually produced synthetically. Exposure to it can cause methemoglobinemia (a blood disorder), convulsions and death.

reticulin

This dermal protein is sometimes used in "cellular" rejuvenation cosmetics.

rhizome

The root-like stem of a plant.

riboflavin

Vitamin B2. See *diet for hair and skin.*

rice bran wax

See *waxes.*

rice powder

A nontoxic ingredient used in face powders.

ricinoleic acid

A *fatty acid* found in castor oil.

Rosa Mosqueta

This is the trade name for *rose hip seed oil* from the *Rosa aff. rubiginosa* (and also the common name for that variety of rose). Rosa Mosqueta has been used for skin burns, cheloids and scars (hypertrophic, hyperchromic and refractile). As a cosmetic, it smoothes wrinkles, *hydrates* the skin and slows new signs of aging. (It's contraindicated for oily skin and acne, however.)

The use of Rosa Mosqueta oil first came to my attention in the summer of 1986, when samples and technical information were sent to me by Dr. Fabiola Carvajal Montiel of the School of Dermatology at the University of Concepción, in Chile. Her case studies were dramatic.

After three months of daily application of Rosa Mosqueta, the wrinkles around the mouth and eyes of one patient were far less noticeable, and some seemed gone entirely. Another female patient with hypertrophic scars on the forehead and around the mouth and eyes showed dramatic improvement after six months of treatment. A 26-year-old male patient had extensive traumatic scars from an operation on his face; after four months of treatment, the scars had almost disappeared.

It's not known whether every type of rose hip seed oil works the same, or if Rosa Mosqueta itself will work for everybody, but it's an excellent skin and hair care treatment (probably due to the *fatty acids* and the *carotenoids* it contains).

Dr. Montiel recommends massaging the Rosa Mosqueta oil in for two or three minutes (to obtain good penetration). I've found that putting a high-quality, fatty-acid-based cream over the Rosa Mosqueta gives even better absorption; however, the cream should be made without petrochemicals (mineral oil, etc.), as these will reduce absorption and affect the skin adversely.

Rosa Mosqueta has no known toxicity. It differs from other herbal oils, having a mild *pH* (around 5.1) and a rather low saponification number. Analyzed extensively by South American researchers, it's been found to be extremely high in *essential fatty acids: linoleic* 41%, linolenic 39% (unsaturated), *oleic* 16%, *palmitic* 3% and *stearic* 0.8% (saturated). Other fatty acids which have been identified are *lauric, myristic* and palmitoleic. The high content of essential fatty acids makes it valuable in the synthesis of *prostaglandins,* which strengthen the immune system and cell membranes, and help tissues grow.

rose hip seed oil

The fruit of the *rose* is called a rose hip (or hipberry). Rose hips contain a lot of *vitamin C* (the concentration varies between 0.24% to 1.25%, depending on ripeness, climate and other factors). They also contain *carotenoids* (at concentrations of 0.01% to 0.05%), flavonoids (0.01% to 0.35%), *pectin* substances (3.4% to 4.6%), polyphenols (2.02% to 2.64%), *fatty acids, glycosides, riboflavin,* sugars and plant acids. Various species of rose hips contain other compounds and demonstrate a wide variety of pharmacological activity. (See *Rosa Mosqueta* for more on this.)

The oil of roses is a light yellow in color and has a strong odor of fresh roses. Rose oils in general can't be synthetically produced, and even a supposedly artificial rose oil must contain some amount of natural rose oil. The scientific study of the rose has been chiefly to improve the odor and the appearance of the flower, rather than the medical or cosmetic uses of the oil.

The FDA considers rose hips (from *Rosa alba L., R. damascena Mill, gallica L.* and their varieties) as safe for use as nutritional or food supplements. To date, rose hip seed oil hasn't been animal tested.

rosemary *(Rosemarinus officinalis)*
Like lavender, rosemary is a major herbal in England and the south of France. Most commercial rosemary oil today comes from France, Spain and Japan. Used in hair tonics for its odor and for its ability to stimulate the *hair bulbs* to renewed activity (it supposedly prevents premature baldness), rosemary oil is also excellent for the skin. Combining rosemary and sage makes an excellent hair rinse and wash.

Smoking rosemary and *coltsfoot* leaves is said to be good for asthma and other problems of the throat and lungs. Queen Elizabeth of Hungary used rosemary oil in her now famous Hungary water, which dates back to 1235. It was made by putting a pound of fresh rosemary tops into a gallon of white wine, and then letting it stand for four days. Queen Elizabeth was partially paralyzed at one time and she is said to have been completely cured by rubbing this water on her arms, legs and feet.

The famous quote from Hamlet—"There's rosemary, that's for remembrance"—is based on the idea that rosemary is good for the brain and the memory. "As for rosemary," Sir Thomas More wrote, "I let it run all over my garden walls, not only because the bees love it, but because it's the herb sacred to remembrance and therefore friendship."

According to *The Treasury of Botany*, rosemary could well be the symbol of women's rights: "There is a vulgar belief in Gloucestershire and other countries that rosemary will not grow well unless the mistress is 'master,' and so touchy are some of the lords of creation upon this point, that we have more than once had reason to suspect them of privately injuring a growing rosemary in order to destroy this evidence for want of authority."

Rosemary was used by the ancients in their religious ceremonies, in place of the more costly incense. In Spain and Italy, it was considered a safeguard against witches and evil. The Spanish revere it because it's one of the bushes that gave shelter to the Virgin Mary, and the Spanish word for it, *romero,* also means *pilgrim.* Rosemary has also been used in the wreath worn by a bride (as a symbol of love and loyalty) and as a New Year's gift.

roses

These prickly bushes or shrubs (family *Rosaceae)* were probably cultivated in Persia and brought to Italy via Mesopotamia, Palestine, Asia Minor and Greece. Horace writes about growing roses in beds, and Pliny advises the deep digging of the soil. Roses were cultivated in ancient Rome and the red rose of Province *(Rosa gallica)* was of Roman origin. There's a Greek myth that the crimson-colored rose sprang from the blood of Adonis. See *rose hip seed oil* and *Rosa Mosqueta.*

rosewater

This aqueous dilution of the essence of roses was first prepared by Avicenna in the 10th century. French rosewater is superior to any developed elsewhere.

royal jelly

This nutritious substance is secreted in the digestive tube of the worker bees. They and the drones eat it for only a few days, but the queen bee eats it her entire life.

Royal jelly contains a full range of *amino acids*, minerals, enzymes and *vitamins A, B, C* and *E*. It has very little cosmetic use, but it's long been a part of Chinese medicine, usually mixed with *tonic* herbs like *astragalus*, codonopsitis and *tang kuei*.

One of the most popular liquid Chinese medicines is ren-shen-feng-wang-jiang, which consists of royal jelly and ginseng. Another Chinese medicine, called ginseng-bee secretion (and sold in Chinese herb shops and some health food stores), contains 12% ginseng, 7% astragalus, 5% deer antler, 5% licorice root, 4% cordyceps, 3% tang kuei , 2% polygonum multiflorum and 2% royal jelly.

rubefacient
In herbology, a substance that produces reddening of the skin and is a mild irritant.

saccharated lime
Used in cosmetics as a preservative and buffer, this chemical is made from oxidated glyconic acid, which is then neutralized with *lime*.

saffron
The dried stigmas of the crocus *(Crocus sativus)* are called saffron. They're used as a deep orange-yellow dye and as an herbal stimulant, antispasmodic and *emmenagogue*.

safrole
See *sassafras*.

salicylic acid
Salicylic acid is the active ingredient in aspirin (whose chemical name is acetylsalicylic acid); it's used in cosmetics at concentrations between 0.025% and 0.2%.

Salicylic acid is an *antipyretic* and *analgesic* that works by inhibiting *prostaglandin* production.

Salicylic acid is absorbed quickly into the body, but secreted slowly. Some countries now forbid its use as a food preservative, and it's not allowed in children's products in the U.S.

Topically, salicylic acid is used as an antiseptic and preservative (as well as for its analgesic and antipyretic properties). Natural wintergreen oil is 98% salicylic acid, and is less likely to burn the skin than pure salicylic acid (see *wintergreen* in the herb chart in Chapter 2).

Although it occurs as an *ester* in several plants, salicylic acid is usually synthesized from *phenol, sodium hydroxide* and carbon dioxide (the first synthesis was achieved by Kolbe in 1874), but the synthetic chemical isn't the same as the plant *esters*. When salicylic acid is heated, it decomposes to *phenol,* which is toxic.

salt

Salts are formed from *acids* by replacing some or all of the hydrogen *ions* with metal ions. There are many different kinds, the best-known of which is sodium chloride (NaCl)—commonly called table salt. Sodium and potassium salts react with *oils* to form soaps.

sambucus

This tree, which grows in temperate climates, has many uses. The oil obtained from the flowers, also known as elder oil, is used in perfumes. The oil of the leaf and bark, as well as the flower water, are used in skin-care creams. The berries are used to make elder-berry wine and elderberry tea.

sandalwood
This extremely expensive oil, derived from a small evergreen tree (genus *Santalum*) of tropical Asia, lends its distinctive fragrance to all kinds of cosmetics. It's also used in Chinese herbal medicine to treat stomach aches, vomiting and gonorrhea.

Coarsely powdering the tree's heartwood and then distilling it with steam or water yields 3% to 5% sandalwood oil. The oil contains 90% or more of alphasantalols and betasantalols, which are responsible for its odor.

saponins
These *sterols* are naturally occurring *glycosides* that foam in water; they're used as foaming, *emulsifying* and detergent agents in cosmetics. Examples are *quillaya bark, yucca* root, soap bark, *soapwort* and *sarsaparilla.*

sarsaparilla
This *saponin* from a plant of of the *Smilax* family may come from Mexico, Central America or South America. It was formerly used to make sweetened carbonated beverages, but was replaced by artificial flavors.

sassafras
The dried bark of this North American tree *(Sassafras albidum)* is used to make an *aromatic* tea with *diaphoretic* and stimulating properties. *Safrole,* the major flavoring ingredient in sassafras, was found to cause cancer in animal tests.

saturated fats
A fat, usually of animal origin, whose *fatty acid* chains can't accomodate any more hydrogen atoms. Compare *unsaturated fats.*

schizonepeta *(Schizonepeta tenuifolia)*
This herb, used in Chinese medicine as a *diaphoretic* and *antipyretic,* is known in China as ching-chieh. It's also used in herbal *tonics* for the skin, to treat pigmentation problems. See *ching-shang.*

scrofula
This is a form of tuberculosis that affects the lymph nodes and also causes inflammation of the joints. Because the disease was formerly associated with filth, poverty and promiscuity, *scrofulous* (affected with scrofula) carried a connotation of moral degeneration.

scute *(Scutellaria baicalensis)*
This herb, known in China as hang-chin, is used for stomach problems and in skin tonics. See *ching-shang.*

sebaceous glands
Glands in the skin that open into *hair follicles* and secrete *sebum.*

sebum
Also known as skin oil, this secretion of the *sebaceous glands* is composed primarily of *fat, keratin* and cellular material.

sedative
In herbology, a substance that has a direct effect on a particular disease.

siler

The root, known as fang-feng in China, is used as an *antipyretic* and *analgesic,* and for skin problems. See *ching-shang.*

SLS

See *sodium lauryl sulfate.*

soapwort

This European perennial herb *(Saponaria officinalis)* has coarse pink or white flowers and leaves that become soapy when bruised. See *saponins.*

sodium

This chemical element (atomic number 11, symbol Na) was named by Sir Humphrey Davy, who isolated it by electrolysis in 1807. The major use of sodium today is in the reduction of animal and vegetable oils into long-chain *fatty alcohols,* which are then used to manufacture soaps and detergents. Sodium can irritate the skin and burn the eyes.

The largest use of sodium (about 60% of the total production) used to be in the manufacture of tetraethyl lead, an antiknock ingredient in gasoline (first introduced by the Ethyl Corporation). Today, however, in order to reduce pollution, leaded gasoline has been largely phased out.

sodium acetate

This allergenic preservative is made by combining *sodium* with acetate (derived from *acetic acid).*

sodium alginate

This natural compound (also known as the salt of *alginic acid)* is used mostly as a thickening agent and *emulsifier* in foods, pharmaceuticals and cosmetics. It isn't known to be toxic.

Sodium alginate is made from algin, a hydrophilic (water-absorbing) substance present in various types of brown algae *(macrocystis, laminaria* and *ascophyllum)*. First the seaweed is prewashed, to leach out undesirable salts; then a dilute *alkaline* solution is used to solubilize the alginic acid present in the seaweed.

sodium alum

This chemical, used as an *astringent, styptic* and *emetic,* is irritating to mucous membranes and may cause allergic reactions. The *alum* used in it is produced by treating bauxite with sulfuric acid to yield alum cake.

sodium ascorbate

This buffered form of *ascorbic acid (vitamin C)* is used in cosmetics as an *antioxidant* and preservative. Like other ascorbates, it can also block the formation of *nitrosamines.*

sodium benzoate

This sodium salt of *benzoic acid* is used as an antiseptic and as a preservative in foods such as soft drinks. There have been allergic reactions to it orally, and it's been listed as moderately toxic due to the *dermatitis* that develops in some people who use it *topically.*

sodium bisulphite

This corrosive synthetic chemical is used as a hair relaxer and a preservative.

sodium borate

This sodium *salt* of *boric acid* is used in cosmetics as an *emulsifier,* preservative and detergent builder.

sodium carbonate

This sodium *salt* of carbonic acid is used in cosmetics as a *humectant* and an *alkalizer.*

sodium citrate
This crystalline *salt* is used in cosmetics as a sequestrant and an *alkalizer,* and in foods as a buffering agent.

sodium fluoride
This sodium *salt* of *fluoride* is added to water in trace amounts to prevent dental caries (cavities). Sodium fluoride can cause mottling of teeth and—if taken orally in high concentrations—death.

sodium hydroxide
Also called caustic soda or *lye,* this corrosive chemical is extremely *alkaline;* an aqueous soluton of just 0.5% (by weight) has a pH of around 12. It's used as an alkalizer and in hair-straightening products; combined with fats, it produces soaps. Also see *potassium hydroxide.*

sodium iodate
This iodine compound has a broad antimicrobial effect. It's used in cosmetics at concentrations of 0.1%, but only in rinse-off products. It's toxic, and irritating to skin and mucous membranes. Dogs were murdered in the lab with 200 mg/kg of it.

sodium lactate
This hygroscopic, viscous, sodium *salt* of *lactic acid* is used as an antacid and as a substitute for *glycerol.*

sodium lauryl sulfate
This very popular ingredient, commonly referred to in the trade as *SLS,* is used as a detergent, *emulsifier* and *surfactant* in over a thousand cosmetic products, including shampoos, toothpastes, lotions and creams. Although you'll find it in many so-called "natural" cosmetics, it's not natural—it's produced synthetically via the Ziegler process and is hardly ever made from coconut oil (even when the label says it is).

SLS is a primary irritant in high concentrations. It's a strong degreaser that dries skin and hair, and has produced skin and hair damage, including cracking of the horny layer of the skin and a severe inflammation of the dermaepidermal tissue.

Reference: "Denaturation of epidermal keratin by surface active agents," *Journal of Investigative Dermatology,* 32:581, 1959.

SLS is frequently combined with *TEA* (triethanolamine), which may be contaminated with the potent carcinogens called *nitrosamines.*

sodium metaphosphate
This term refers to several crystalline, sodium *salts* of metaphosphoric acid that are used in cosmetics as *emulsifiers* or texturizers.

sodium palmitate
This sodium *salt* of *palmitic acid* is used in cosmetics as a texturizer.

sodium PCA
This chemical, sometimes abbreviated *NaPCA,* is a sodium *salt* of pyroglutamic acid. A few years ago, it was a popular buzzword in cosmetics, with advertising copy describing it as a substance in our own skins that can remoisturize the skin from the outside in. However, synthetic NaPCA can cause strong allergic reactions when applied *topically,* and can severely dry the skin by absorbing moisture from it.

sodium pyrrithione
This toxic chemical, used in cosmetics at 250 to 1000 *ppm,* can cause allergic reactions. Lab rats have been murdered with it at 875 mg/kg, and mice at 1172 mg/kg. First synthesized in 1948, it's a cyclic thiohydroxamic acid and a *pyridine* derivative. Trade names include Sodium Omadine and Pyrion-Na.

sodium salicylate

This sodium *salt* of *salicylic acid,* used as a sun filter, antiseptic and preservative, can cause allergic reactions, especially in people allergic to aspirin.

sodium thioglycolate

Like all *thioglycolate* compounds, this chemical, used in permanents as a hair relaxer, is a primary irritant.

solid extracts

Solid extracts are thin to thick liquids or semisolids prepared from *native extracts* and diluted to the appropriate strength. Also known as pilular extracts, they're usually the same strength as powdered extracts.

sorbic acid

This *organic acid,* used in cosmetic creams and lotions as an antifungal preservative, is toxic. (Don't confuse it with sorbitol, a natural *humectant.)* Its trade name is Sentry.

First isolated in 1859 by A. F. Hofmann from the berries of the mountain ash (in the form of parasorbic acid), today it's synthesized by condensing crotonaldehyde and malonic acid in a *pyridine* solution.

sorbitan laurate, oleate, palmitate, stearate, etc.

These cosmetic ingredients, used as *nonionic surfactants, humectants,* binders and *emulsifiers,* can cause allergic reactions. They're made from *lauric acid* and *sorbitol* compounds.

sorbitol

This crystalline, slightly sweet *alcohol,* occurring naturally in the mountain ash *(Sorbus acuparia)* but usually produced industrially by a reduction reaction of D-glucose, is used in cosmetics as a *humectant,* binder, *plasticizer* and softener.

soybean (or soy) oil
This pale yellow oil, consisting mostly of *glycerides* of *linoleic, oleic,* linolenic and *palmitic acids,* is used in cosmetics as an *emollient.*

spermaceti
This oil, derived from sperm whales, has been illegal to use in any products in the United States since 1971, when the Marine Mammal Protection Act was passed. See *waxes.*

spermatorrhea
The involuntary discharge of semen without sexual intercourse.

squalene
There are recent claims that this *saturated hydrocarbon* bolsters the immune system, increases oxygenation, improves metabolism and strengthens the liver. Although squalene is typically obtained from shark liver oil, the identical chemical can be derived from olives, and you don't have to kill sharks to get it. Olive oil squalene is cheaper to produce, more stable against *oxidation,* of a higher food grade (due to its vegetarian source), purer and more compatible with the skin than shark-derived squalene (or, for that matter, than *lanolin).*

staphylococcus
This gram-positive bacteria may contaminate cosmetics.

stearalkonium chloride
This *quaternary ammonium* compound is used almost universally in hair conditioners, both those that are mass-merchandised and so-called "natural" ones. It was originally developed by the textile industry for use as a fabric softener, and it also has antistatic proper-

ties. These characteristics are important in a hair conditioner only if you think of your hair as a ball of yarn. If you think of it as protein that grows out of living tissue, then you'll avoid this chemical.

stearate
An *ester* of *stearic acid.*

steareth-2, -4, -7, -10, -20 and -30
These polyethylene *glycol* ethers of *stearyl alcohol* are used as *emollients* and *emulsifiers.* They're synthetic chemicals that can cause allergic reactions.

stearic acid
This waxy, crystalline, *fatty acid* is typically derived from tallow and other animal fats, but it's also found in *cocoa butter* and other hard vegetable fats. Used in cosmetics as a base and an *emollient,* it can cause some allergic reactions.

stearyl alcohol
This *fatty alcohol* is found in whale, porpoise and dolphin oils, but it's usually produced by *hydrogenating* *stearic acid.* It's used similarly to *cetyl alcohol.*

steroids
These fat-soluble compounds, which occur naturally but can also be synthesized, include *sterols,* sex *hormones,* adrenal hormones, bile acids and some cancer-stimulating hydrocarbons.

sterols
This class of usually *unsaturated* solid *alcohols* is widely distributed in the fatty tissues of animals and plants. *Cholesterol* is a sterol. Also see *steroids.*

stilbene dyes
These yellow to orange dyes or fluorescent brighteners are derived from an *aromatic hydrocarbon* called stilbene.

stillingia oil
This pale yellow drying oil is obtained from the seeds of the Chinese tallow tree *(Sapium sebiferum* or *Stillingia sebifera).*

stimulant
Any substance that quickens physiological activity.

stomachic
In herbology, a substance that strengthens and tones the stomach.

stramonium
This chemical, which is similar to belladonna, is used in cosmetics for its antiperspirant properties, but it's lethal if ingested. Derived from the dried leaf of the thorn apple (genus *Datura),* it contains the *alkaloids* atropine, lyoscyamine and scopolamine, and is used as an asthma medicine.

stratum corneum
The outer, horny layer of the *epidermis.*

strength of extracts
The potency of botanical drug extracts is generally expressed in two ways. If the active ingredient is known, the concentration of that is given; otherwise, the concentration of the crude drug is given. In that case, a strength of 1:4 means that one part of extract is equivalent to, or derived from, four parts of crude drug.

strontium hydroxide
This *alkaline* solid is used to make soaps and greases and in refining beet sugar. A synthetic chemical, it's an irritant.

styptic
This term can refer to either a plant that contracts organic tissue (that is, an *astringent)* or to one that stops bleeding (that is, a *hemostatic,* like *alum* or tannin).

subcutaneous
Under the skin.

succinic acid
This acid, which occurs naturally in amber, lignite, *turpentine,* animal fluids and elsewhere, is used in cosmetics as an antiseptic, buffer and neutralizer.

sulfate
This synthetic liquid, made with sulfated oils, is used to make synthetic soaps and detergents like *sodium lauryl sulfate* (a chemical used in soaps, detergents and shampoo). Sulfates are harmful to marine life and the environment. They can cause allergic reactions and dry skin and hair, and can irritate the eyes.

sulfated oils
These oils or *fatty acids,* treated with sulfuric acid or oleum to make them water-soluble, are used as wetting and *emulsifying* agents.

sulfites
See *bisulfites.*

sulfur
This chemical element (atomic number 16, symbol S) was discovered prior to recorded history. Its elemental character was first recorded by the pioneering French chemist Lavoisier in 1777. Two main types of compounds are made with sulfur—sulfides and oxides.

sunlight
See *ultraviolet rays.*

surface-active
Capable of reducing the *surface tension* of a liquid. The noun is *surfactant.*

surface tension
The property of a liquid that makes its surface resemble a stretched elastic membrane. Surface tension is what allows you to fill a glass of water so that it bulges slightly above the lip. *Surfactants* reduce surface tension.

surfactant
A substance that reduces the *surface tension* of a liquid in which it's dissolved. The adjective is *surface-active.*

tang-kuei *(Angelica sinensis)*
This root is used in China as a sedative, analgesic, *emmenagogue* and for skin pigmentation problems. See *tang-kuei-shao-yao-san.*

tang-kuei-shao-yao-san
This Chinese herbal mixture is used for pigmentation problems that occur primarily in pale complexions (e.g. freckles and melasma), for various body pains, and to improve circulation. The formula for it is one part alisma, one part *atractylodes,* one part *cnidium,* one part *coix,* one part peony and one part *tang-kuei.* (Chinese

herbal tonics should come to no more than a total weight of sixteen ounces, unless otherwise stated.)

tannic acid
Formerly used to treat burns, this complex *phenolic* acid is now used medically as an *astringent,* and industrially for tanning, dyeing and making ink. It's found in plants such as powdered gallnuts, shredded tara, quebracho wood, chestnut wood, wattle, sumac and valonia.

tar oil
This *volatile* oil, used in cosmetics as an antiseptic and deodorant, is distilled from wood tar (usually pine).

tartaric acid
Used in cosmetics as a buffer, and sometimes to neutralize *permanent wave* solutions, this *acid* is found in fresh fruit. In strong concentrations, it may irritate the skin.

TEA *(triethanolamine)*
This synthetic chemical is used ubiquitously—both in mass-merchandised and so-called "natural" cosmetics—as a *pH* adjuster, an *emulsifier* and a preservative, and to make *fatty acid* soaps. A combination of *ammonia* and ethylene oxide, this amino alcohol may be contaminated with nitrosamines, which are potent carcinogens. See *nitrosamines.*

TEA-lauryl sulfate
This very popular shampoo ingredient, used as a synthetic detergent, *emulsifier* and *surfactant,* is a combination of triethanolamine *(TEA)* and the *salt* of lauryl sulfuric acid. It should be avoided, since it may be con-

taminated with *nitrosamines* (because of the TEA) and because it's drying to the skin and hair.

tea tree oil

In 1770, Lieutenant (soon-to-be Captain) Cook of the British Royal Navy came across the tree *Melaleuca alternifolia,* which grows only in the northeastern corner of Australia. He brewed a spicy tea from its leaves, from which the plant gets its common name—the tea tree. (The tea tree is no relation to the varieties of camellia from whose leaves we brew the black tea and green tea we commonly drink.) Sir Joseph Banks, a botanist with the expedition, brought samples of tea tree leaves back to England with him.

Today, tea tree oil is used as an antiseptic and germicide; in those applications, it's thought to be many times stronger than carbolic acid. It also can be used for insect bites, for skin problems and as a dentifrice and mouthwash. Due to its strong odor, it's not often used in cosmetics, but if it's mixed with other *essential oils* to compensate for the odor, it can be used in dandruff shampoos, face masks and *topical* creams.

Mentioned in the *British Pharmacoepia* (1949), tea tree oil should conform to the Australian standard of a terpinen-4 ol content of at least 30%, with 15% cineole.

terpineol

This monoterpene *alcohol* is used in soaps and perfumes for its fragrance—one variety smells like hyacinths, another like lilacs. It's usually obtained from pine oil (although it occurs in many herbal *essential oils).*

tetrabromo-o-cresol

This *phenolic* compound used in deodorants and shampoos comes from cresol, a poisonous isometric phenol occurring in *coal tar* (it's synthesized by bromination of o-cresol). A primary skin irritant, it's also used in the manufacture of anti-knock gasoline. Its trade name is Rabulen-TI.

tetrasodium EDTA

Used in cosmetics as a sequestering agent, this chemical is an eye and skin irritant.

theobroma oil

Another name for cocoa oil or cocoa butter, used in cosmetics as an *emollient*. See *cocoa butter*.

thimerosal

This toxic chemical is a common preservative in contact lens solutions. Studies in Sweden have shown that a high percentage of people are allergic to it, and the European Economic Community has limited its use to eye makeup, requiring that any products using it bear the warning: *Contains thimerosal*. It's an organic mercurial anionic, and mercurial compounds are deadly poisons. Its trade names are Merfamin, Merthiolate and Merzonin.

thioglycolates

These strong-smelling chemical compounds are used for permanent waves (mainly in the form of an ammonium salt) and as depilatory agents (in the form of a calcium or other salt). The smell comes from a reaction between chloroacetic acid and hydrogen sulfide.

Thioglycolates work by breaking the chemical bonds of the hair. In depilatories, they turn the hair into a gummy mass that can be washed away; in permanent wave solutions, they're not supposed to have the same effect, of course, although the same chemicals are used.

If ingested, thioglycolate compounds are toxic in small doses. Corrosive and irritating, they damage the hair and skin, as well as any metal and fabric they come in contact with. The damage is increased by the *surfactants* usually included in permanent wave solutions, which remove oils from the skin and hair in order to optimize penetration of the thioglycolates.

Worse yet, many surfactants anesthetize the eyeball, so if any thioglycolate (or other harmful chemical compound) gets into the eye, the burn won't be felt until substantial damage has already occurred. For these reasons, permanent wave products should be avoided. Also see *permanent waves.*

thioindigoid
This class of dyes is similar to *indigo.*

threonine
An *essential amino acid.*

thymol
This crystalline *phenol* is used as a *fungicide,* antifungal, preservative, fragrance and flavoring. It occurs naturally in thyme and many other *essential oils,* and is also manufactured synthetically.

tincture
A tincture is an alcoholic or hydroalcoholic (water and alcohol) solution that usually contains the active principles of botanicals in comparatively low concentrations.

titanium dioxide

This white powder is used as a pigment in eye make-up, sunscreens and foundation makeup (both powdered and liquid). It's also used as an *opacifying agent,* for its covering power, brilliance and reflectivity. An *inorganic salt* that's also used in house paint, enamels, plastics, paper products and shoe whiteners, titanium dioxide shouldn't be inhaled.

tocopherol

Another name for *vitamin E,* a fat-soluble *antioxidant* that's used as a preservative in the oil phase of cosmetics.

toilet water

Also known as *eau de toilette,* toilet water has a less concentrated fragrance (4–8%) and a lower-grade alcohol (80%) than perfume.

toluene

This *aromatic* liquid *hydrocarbon* (similar to *benzene)* is used as a solvent in cosmetics, especially nail polishes, and also in dyes, in pharmaceuticals and as a blending agent for gasoline. Produced commercially from petrochemicals, it's toxic and narcotic in high concentrations.

tonic

In herbology, a substance that strengthens and stimulates the system.

topical

Applied to the skin.

tragacanth
This herbal gum is used as a thickener in cosmetics and in hair care products as a hairspray or setting-lotion ingredient. Also see *gums*.

trichloroethane
This *hydrocarbon* used in cosmetics as a solvent, has irritating, narcotic vapors, and may be fatal if inhaled, ingested or absorbed through the skin. Don't confuse it with *trichloroethylene*.

trichloroethylene
Used in *astringent* formulations, this *hydrocarbon* is a known irritant and carcinogen. Don't confuse it with *trichloroethane*.

trichology
The scientific study of the hair.

triclocarban
This toxic chemical, which can cause allergic and pho-tosensitization reactions, is the most commonly used *antibacterial* agent in deodorant soaps (in concentrations of 1% to 2%); it's also used in antiperspirants and skin-cleansing products. Because triclocarban kills some—but not all—bacteria, it can cause an imbalance in the bacterial flora that surrounds the body.

Triclocarban is absorbed through the skin—one study lists absorption at around 14%—and the long-term consequences of this are unknown. It isn't allowed to be used in maternity units or on infants, as cases of methemoglobinemia have been reported.

Triclocarban is a carbanilide compound prepared from 3,4-dichloraniline and 4-chlor-ophenylisocyanate.

triclosan
This *bactericide* is a common ingredient in deodorants and deodorant soaps. Although it has shown low oral toxicity and has been approved by the *FDA*, absorption through the skin (which is clearly a factor in a soap that's used over the entire body) may cause liver damage.

trideceth-3, -6, -10, *etc.*
These compounds are used in cosmetics as *emulsifiers* and binders. Polyethylene glycol *ethers* of tridecyl alcohol, they're made from *paraffin,* a *mineral oil* product.

triethanolamine
See *TEA.*

triphenylmethane dye *(tritan)*
See *colors.*

tryptophan
By stimulating the production of serotonin, a neurotransmitter, the *amino acid* L-tryptophan is said to help you relax and sleep. Because one batch of triptophan used in food supplement tablets was found to be contaminated years ago, the FDA has banned the importation of all triptophan.

turkey-red oil
Used in shampoos since the 1880s, this sulfated castor oil was the first synthetic detergent. It's effective in hard or soft water, but it doesn't foam much and tends to strip color from the hair.

turpentine

This natural *hydrocarbon,* used in cosmetics as a solvent, is isolated from pine trees. It irritates skin and mucous membranes and may cause allergic reactions.

turtle oil

This oil, obtained from the giant sea turtle *Chelonium,* is used as an *emollient.* It's no better than a good vegetable oil, but it destroys an endangered species. This is another example of advertising creating a demand for an unethical product.

Tweens

Trade name for the *polysorbates.*

2,4-dichlorobenzyl alcohol

This alcohol, used in combination with *bronopol* and *Germall 115,* is toxic and a danger to the environment. Its trade names are Dybenal and Myacide SP.

2-naphthol

See *1-naphthol.*

tyrosine

Because this *amino acid* participates in the production of *melanin,* it's used in cosmetics to increase the tanning effect on the skin.

ultraviolet rays

These rays (also known as *UV)* have wave lengths shorter than visible light and longer than x-rays. *(Ultraviolet* means *beyond violet*—violet being at the top end of visible light's color spectrum.)

Overexposure to ultraviolet radiation will damage the skin over time and can cause skin cancer, so a sunblock with SPF 15 is advisable. (SPF stands for *sun protection factor.* An SPF of 15 means that you can spend 15 hours in the sun with—presumably—no more damage than if you spend one hour in the sun without it.) The best protection is provided by UV-absorbers *(PABA* is a good one) and UV-reflectors *(titanium dioxide* is a good one).

umbelliferone

A natural *phenol* found in many plants, such as galbanum or asafetida.

undecylenic acid

Used as an antidandruff agent in shampoos (in a concentration of 1%), this *organic acid* is somewhat similar to the acid in our own perspiration. Nevertheless, it's a primary skin irritant and a toxic chemical that has murdered lab rats at 2.5 g/kg.

A *zinc* salt, its chemical name is undecylenic acid monoethanolamide-di-sodium-sulfosuccinate. It's sold under the trade names of Declid, Renselin and Sevinon.

unsaturated fats

A fat, usually of vegetable origin, whose *fatty acid* chains can accommodate more hydrogen atoms. Compare *saturated fats.*

urea

This end product of normal mammalian metabolism, found in urine and other body fluids, is a white, crystalline or powdery, water-soluble compound. It's used medically as a *diuretic,* and is sometimes used in cosmetics.

When combined with *formaldehyde,* urea becomes a syrup. Mixed with cellulose and coloring matter, that syrup is used to treat textiles and in laminating. Many people are allergic to fabrics that contain urea-formaldehyde, and anyone allergic to *ammonia* will probably be allergic to urea. It's also dangerous to use products containing urea around the eyes.

Because of its high nitrogen content, urea is also used to manufacture fertilizer. Commercially, it's manufactured by the partial hydrolysis of cyanamide, and by heating carbon dioxide and ammonia under pressure. In 1828, F. Wholer prepared urea from phosgene and ammonia, by rearrangement of ammonium cyanate.

uric acid

Sometimes used in cosmetics instead of *allantoin* or *comfrey* extracts, which are superior ingredients, this is a nitrogenous compound that's present in the urine of most mammals. Elevated uric acid is believed to be a symptom of gout.

usnic acid

This antibiotic is used in anti-acne formulas at concentrations of 0.1%–0.3% and in deodorants at concentrations of 0.2%. It's also used as a local therapeutic agent.

Usnic acid is a toxic chemical that's been used to murder lab rats at 30 mg/kg and mice at 25 mg/kg, and it's showed subcutaneous toxicity to mice at 700 mg/kg. It's produced naturally by lichens *(Cladonia stellaris, Usnea barbata* and others).

UV rays

See *ultraviolet rays.*

vasoconstrictor
A substance that narrows blood vessels, thus raising blood pressure.

vasodilator
A substance that dilates (widens) blood vessels, thus lowering blood pressure.

vegan
A person who eats, or a diet that contains, no animal products of any kind—that is, no milk, cheese, eggs, etc.

vegetable gums
See *gums*.

vermifuge
A substance that destroys intestinal worms.

vermilion
This red pigment, whose color varies from crimson to nearly orange, is used primarily as an artist's color and in rubber. Its name comes from *vermiculus,* Latin for *small worm,* because it was originally made from *cochineal*, a red dye obtained by crushing the bodies of dried, worm-like insects.

Vermilion was also derived from the mineral cinnabar, but it's now synthesized from a reaction involving *mercury, sulfur* and *sodium hydroxide.* Because it contains mercury, synthesized vermillion is toxic, but it's still used as a coloring agent in some cosmetics. Another name for synthesized vermillion is mercuric sulfide.

vesicant
A substance that produces blisters.

vetiver oil

This oil, which is used in perfumes, cosmetics and soaps, is obtained from khuskhus *(Andropogon zizamoides),* an *aromatic* grass from India.

vinegar

This sour liquid is used in cosmetics as a solvent or *pH* adjuster. Vinegar contains around 4% or 5% *acetic acid,* and may irritate the skin if used in concentrations that are too strong.

vitamin A

This fat-soluble vitamin, whose deficiency causes night-blindness, may have more cosmetic uses than any other vitamin. As a preservative, the oil from carrots, which is high in vitamin A and provitamin A, has been used with great success, in combination with *vitamin C, vitamin E* and *grapefruit seed* extract.

Vitamin A helps remedy rough and dry skin (including mucous membranes) and has also been used in the treatment of *psoriasis.* A daily intake of 50,000 units of vitamin A and 50 mg of *zinc* has reportedly cleared some forms of acne, and a version of vitamin A—retinoic acid (RA), also called vitamin A acid (which is classified as a drug)—has been used as a *topical* acne treatment as well, though some people are allergic to it. It's also been used to treat aging skin (RA causes the shedding of skin cells).

Vitamin A can be obtained from fish liver oil, liver, carrots, green and yellow vegetables, eggs, milk and dairy products, margarine and yellow fruits. As an *antioxidant,* it prevents vitamin C from being *oxidized* too quickly in the body. Some studies have found that amounts of vitamin A over 100,000 units daily over a period of months can be toxic, but normal dosages are harmless.

vitamin B complex
These water-soluble vitamins include B1 (thiamine), B2 *(riboflavin)*, B3 (niacin), B5 *(pantothenic acid* and panthenol), B6 (pyridoxine), B12 (cyanocobalamin), *biotin,* folic acid, *PABA* (para-aminobenzoic acid), carnitine, choline and *inositol.* Individual B vitamins are used in various cosmetics.

vitamin C
An *antioxidant,* vitamin C *(ascorbic acid)* can preserve cosmetics both in the water phase and—particularly in its fat-soluble form, ascorbyl palmitate—in the oil phase as well. It plays an essential role in building *collagen,* the connective tissue that holds us together. Vitamin C occurs in fresh foods, especially citrus fruits, along with a complex of other factors (rutin, hesperidin and other bioflavonoids) that help promote its effectiveness and build capillary strength.

vitamin D
This fat-soluble vitamin, chemically related to the *steroids,* is essential for healthy bones and teeth and for the absorption of *calcium.* The body can produce its own vitamin D if the skin is exposed to the sun (with certain natural oils present).

vitamin E
One of the most potent natural, fat-soluble *antioxidants* in use—particularly when combined with *vitamin C* and *vitamin A*—vitamin E is used in cosmetics as a preservative. Only 100 to 200 parts per million of vitamin E are needed to provide stability and to protect

the oil phase of *emollients,* moisturizers, lotions and creams (and easily *oxidized* substances like vitamin A and *saturated* oils) from oxidation.

Vitamin E may be natural or synthetic depending on the isomer and manufacturer; if natural, it's from vegetable sources. The *D* isomer generally only occurs naturally, although it can be isolated from a synthetic vitamin E; a *DL* prefix indicates the vitamin E is synthetic. Look for the NSVEA (Natural Source Vitamin E Association) label on vitamin E supplements.

vitamin F
See *essential fatty acids.*

vitiligo
This skin abnormality is characterized by areas with loss of pigment surrounded by deeply pigmented borders.

volatile
Something that evaporates readily at normal temperatures and pressures.

walnut extract
This extract from the husk of the walnut *(Juglans regia)* is superior to artificial hair coloring chemicals. It dyes hair a natural deep-brown color, and it can be combined with *henna* and coffee to make a deep red-brown.

waxes
Waxes (which can be white, brown, green, yellow, amber or black) have many cosmetic, food and industrial uses. Their use in cosmetics can be traced back to ancient Egypt, where women coated their bodies with a mixture of melted wax and *essential oils.* They would then attend a festive occasion (perhaps a religious cer-

emony) and, as they danced, the wax would slowly melt, releasing the fragrance of the essential oils.

Another ancient use for waxes is to create *emulsions* for cosmetic creams. The Greek physician Galen (who worked in Rome around 150 A.D.) used beeswax in the first cold cream. Today, however, synthetic and petroleum waxes are more frequently used than vegetable or animal ones. (Vegetable waxes—also called plant waxes—are *esters* of *fatty acids* and *fatty alcohols.)*

An *aesthetician* might use a wax as a skin care mask or to increase absorption of other skin care products into the skin (a process called hydro-occlusion). For example, there's a treatment in which arthritis medication is combined with hot wax and then spread over the hand, providing therapeutic results as it cools. Here are some of the waxes commonly used in cosmetics:

Beeswax is excreted by the honeybee, *Apis mellifera* (family *Apidae)* to construct its honeycomb. It's extracted by boiling the honeycomb in water and skimming the wax off the top. The color of beeswax varies from deep brown to light amber, depending on what flowers the bee visited for pollen. Beeswax is compatible with most other waxes, fatty acids, fatty alcohols and plant glycerides. Some people are allergic to it.

Bayberry wax is gray-green and is very *aromatic*. It's obtained by boiling the wax-coated berries of the bayberry shrub and skimming off the wax as it floats to the top. The bayberry shrub grows in the coastal areas of North, Central and South America, but most commercial bayberry wax comes from Columbia. Its melting point is 100°–120° F, and it's compatible with most other waxes, fatty acids, *hydrocarbons* and plant glycerides.

Candelilla wax is found in the scales covering reed-like plants *(Euphorbiea antisiphilitica, Euphorbiea cerifera* and *Pedilanthus pavonis)* that grow wild on rocky slopes and plains in northwest Mexico and southern Texas. When the plant is boiled in water with a small amount of sulfuric acid, the light brown to yellow wax floats to the top and can be skimmed off. This wax isn't as hard as *carnauba,* and it takes several days to reach its maximum hardness. Its melting point is 155°–162° F, and it's compatible with all vegetable and animal waxes and some hydrocarbons.

Carnauba wax is exuded by the leaves of a Brazilian tree *(Copernica cerifera)* to conserve its moisture. The natives of Brazil use various products from this tree for many necessities, which is why they call it *arbol del vida,* which means *tree of life.* There are many carnauba palms in other parts of South America, Ceylon and equatorial Africa, but only the Brazilian trees have the wax (the result of Brazil's irregular rainy seasons). Yellow in color, carnauba wax melts at 181° F and higher, and it's compatible with all vegetable, animal and mineral waxes as well as with many plant glycerides, fatty acids and hydrocarbons.

Ceresin wax, a petroleum product that's derived from the mineral ozokerite by refining and bleaching, is considered a higher-grade *paraffin.* White to tan in color, its melting point is 128°–150° F, and it's compatible with vegetable, animal and mineral waxes, many synthetic chemical resins, fatty acids, plant glycerides and hydrocarbons.

Japan wax is a pale, cream-colored vegetable wax with a gummy feel, obtained from the berries of several Japanese sumac (hazel) trees. The berries are aged, then crushed to get at the wax-coated kernels inside; the wax is extracted by pressure or with a solvent. To refine it, it's melted and filtered, then bleached with chemicals or sunlight. Its melting point is 115°–120°F, and it's compatible with beeswax, *cocoa butter* and plant glycerides.

Jojoba wax is made by *hydrogenating* the liquid wax of the jojoba shrub *(Simmondsia chinensis)* with a nickel-copper catalyst at mild temperatures and pressures. The hard, white wax that results melts at 149°–154° F, and is compatible with most other waxes and plant glycerides.

Microcrystalline wax is a mixture of hydrocarbons and paraffins in a matrix of small crystals. Colored white, yellow and black, its melting point is 140–205°F, and it's compatible with most other waxes.

Montan wax is a dark-brown, brown or tan wax derived from lignites (low-grade coal) from Central Europe and California. They're crushed to a powder and the waxy material is extracted by solvents. Montan wax melts at 181°–190°F, and it's compatible with vegetable waxes, hydrocarbons and *resins.*

Ouricury wax is exuded from the leaves of the ouricury palm *(Syagrus coronata)* which grows in Brazil. The greenish-brown wax can only be removed by scraping the leaves with a sharp instrument. The color varies depending on the care taken during processing. It melts at 180°–184° F, and is compatible with all vegetable, animal and mineral waxes, resins, fatty acids, plant glycerides and hydrocarbons.

Ozokerite wax is a bituminous product occurring near petroleum deposits in Poland, Austria, Russia, Ukraine, Utah and Texas. Unlike the paraffins and microcrystalline waxes, ozokerite waxes have long fibers. As a hydrocarbon product, this wax is less desirable in cosmetics. Ozokerite comes in white and yellow, and its melting point varies according to grade (most flakes melt at 152°–165° F). It's compatible with all vegetable waxes, resins, animal waxes, plant glycerides and fatty acids.

Paraffin waxes are hard, white, crystalline materials refined from petroleum by the use of various solvents. They're very widely used in cereal wraps, food wraps, corrugated containers, cheese and vegetable coatings, candles and textiles. If you want to avoid petrochemicals, paraffin is one of the substances that will make doing that the most difficult.

Normally white in color, paraffins take on a dark color (and begin to smell) when they become *rancid.* Paraffins melt at between 112° and 165° F, and are compatible with some vegetable, mineral and animal waxes.

Rice bran is a commercially important source of edible oil, and this oil contains a wax that's removed by purification and crystallization. The resulting *rice bran wax* is better as a coating for fruits, vegetables, confectionery and chewing gum than paraffins or petrochemical waxes, and it's also suitable for cosmetics. Varying from tan to light brown in color, it melts between 169° and 181° F. It's compatible with all other waxes, fatty acids, plant glycerides and hydrocarbons.

Spermaceti wax comes from the sperm whale, whose murder is forbidden by U.S. government regulations. See *spermaceti.*

wetting agents
These substances promote the penetration or spreading of a liquid, and are used to help mix solids with liquids. See *humectant.*

wheat bran
This fibrous outer coating of the wheat kernel is used in masks and baths for its calming and exfoliating effect.

wheat germ oil
Used in cosmetics as a moisturizer, this oil from the embryo of the wheat kernel is high in *vitamin E.*

white camellia *(Camellia oleifera Abel)*
The oil expressed from the seeds of the camellia flower is an excellent hair and skin *emollient,* high in *essential fatty acids.* A *green tea* made from the leaves is also used in hair care and skin care products. Wild white camellia has been used for hundreds of years in China and Japan. I first brought it to the United States from the Longevity Village in China, to use as a cosmetic ingredient in a variety of skin and hair care products. See *wild white camellia* in the herb chart in Chapter 2.

whitehead
A small, whitish mass beneath the surface of the skin caused by the retention of *sebum.* See *blackhead.*

white lead
Beginning in Elizabethan times, women used this highly toxic substance (also called ceruse) to give their faces a smooth porcelain finish. Around 1900, it was finally replaced by rice powder.

wood alcohol
See *methanol.*

xanthan gum
See *gums*.

xanthene dyes
Used to dye textiles and paper, and for fluorescent effects, this group of bright yellow to pink to blue-red dyes is distinguished by their xanthene nucleus. When used in cosmetics, they should be avoided, since they can cause *phototoxicity.* See *colors.*

xylenol
This *phenol* compound, a petroleum distillate, is used as a disinfectant and to make phenolic *resins.*

xylitol
This sugar is derived from the cell walls of plants, especially straw, corncobs, oat hulls, cottonseed hulls and wood.

yarrow
This herb is used as an *astringent.* See the herb chart in Chapter 2.

yeast
Fungi that produce enzymes and convert sugar to *alcohol* and carbon dioxide, yeasts are a dietary source of the B vitamin folic acid. Also see *brewer's yeast.*

ylang-ylang oil
This fragrant oil, obtained from flowers in the Philippines, is used in perfumes and as a flavoring in food. It can cause some allergic reactions. See the herb chart in Chapter 2.

zinc

Fourth among all metals produced industrially (after iron, copper and aluminum), zinc's largest use is as a protective coating for other metals. It's also present in our bodies; for example, men's hair contains 212 mg/kg of zinc, and women's hair contains 116 mg/kg.

Zinc has a variety of pharmaceutical uses. Taking 20 mg a day is said to help some cases of acne, and children with a skin disease called acrodermatitis enteropathica (which causes lesions on the skin, poor nutrient absorption, bowel problems, and stunted growth) have also found relief with zinc supplements—taking 35 mg daily cleared up the skin and corrected the bowel problems.

In addition, zinc ointment is said to clear up dandruff. It isn't the best form of dandruff therapy, however, since it leaves a white, gummy residue in the hair.

zinc oxide

This white powder is used in ointments to protect the skin from *ultraviolet rays* and to treat diaper rash. It's also used for its *astringent* properties, and as a pigment in pharmaceutical and cosmetic products. Occurring in nature as zincite, it's a white solid that isn't soluble in water.

zinc pyrrithione

This toxic chemical is found in gels, creams, talcum powder and shampoos at concentrations of 100 to 250 *ppm*. A cyclic thiohydroxamic acid, it's a primary skin irritant. Its trade names are Zinc Omadine and Vancide.

Chapter 2
A chart of useful herbs

What do arnica, betulla, ivy, horse chestnut and bladderwrack have in common? Betulla sounds a bit fattening, like something you don't want to happen to your hips, but if you call it by its common name—birch—then it sounds slim and trim, and that's exactly how it's used.

Spas in Europe use a mixture of betulla and the other herbs listed above in whirlpool baths designed to sweat away the pounds, and some cosmetic manufacturers put them in anticellulite creams, which are often put under plastic wraps to squeeze away the pounds.

Does this mixture work? There is a temporary displacement of liquid build-up in the fat cells, but it's probably far more successful if a workout program goes along with it.

The ancient Greeks called fennel *marathon* (from *maraino—to grow thin),* because the seeds, leaves and roots were used in drinks for weight loss.

Did you know that the seeds of the *hips* (fruits) of a variety of rose known as Rosa Mosqueta® can reduce wrinkles and help burns and even make some scars disappear?

Maybe you've heard that licorice root has a substance in it known as glycyrahizinic acid which is being used as an alternate treatment to boost the immune system in AIDS patients.

Not everybody needs to know that two substances found in camomile—chamazulene and d-gaiacturonic acid—are antimicrobial, but it is good to know that camomile can be valued not only as a skin emollient and normalizer, but has other uses as well.

How many men have been told that the juice from the common nettle contains phytosterols that are believed to stimulate hair growth?

Some substances found in herbs are tongue-twisters like (2)-5-tetradecen-14-olide. Just because the name is a tongue-twister doesn't mean it's some synthetic chemical. (2)-5-tetradecen-14-olide is what gives the unique, musky odor to ambrette seeds.

(2)-5-tetradecen-14-olide provides a way for us to enjoy this fragrance without killing a musk ox. There are other lovely musk fragrances in herbs—which is good news for animal lovers who don't want animals harmed in lab experiments or in order to create a cosmetic or perfume.

The purpose of the chart that takes up the rest of this chapter is to map the various uses of herbs for the hair and skin. (If you run across any terms you don't know, look them up in Chapter 1.) I've detailed uses from folk medicine and added my own comments about various things I've discovered in working with these herbs. I hope you find the chart useful.

Herb name, synonyms, folk use	Parts used — Extracts	Typical substances	Cosmetic use	Properties and other uses	Similar plants	Comments
ABSINTHIUM (*Artemisia absinthium*) SYN: Wormwood, Absinthe, Armoise FOLK MEDICINE: Used as aromatic bitter for anorexia and as digestive tonic for gall bladder disorders.	Leaves & flowering tops — Glycolic	Volatile oil, azulene, thujone, pinene, camphene, thojyl alcohol, absinthin, ketopelenolide, carotene (0.05%), ascorbic acid (0.26%), tannins (7.7%), essential oils.	Oil used as fragrance in soaps, creams, lotions, perfumes	Bitter tonic, Emmenagogue, flavor for vermouth (0.024%). Maximum use in food is about 0.006%	Wormseed and other Artemisia species. Marijuana (similar psychological effect because of the thujone & tetrahydrocannabinol).	In perfumes: maximum 0.25%; in soaps, 0.01%. Approved by FDA for food if thujone-free. Average maximum amount used 0.024%.
ACACIA (*Acacia senegal*) Gum Arabic, Egyptian thorn	Stems & branches — Gum	Sugars, acids (glucuronics), calcium, magnesium, potassium, sodium	Used in hairsprays, wavesets, & as a thickener.	Demulcent, mucilage, suspending & emulsifying. Trochisci, syrups, jujubes.	Gum tragacanth, kordofan gum, mogadore gum, Indian gum, quince seeds.	1 to 4 drachms of gum creates a syrup. Gum can be dissolved in water.

Herb name, synonyms, folk use	Parts used — Extracts	Typical substances	Cosmetic use	Properties and other uses	Similar plants	Comments
ACONITE *(Aconitum napellus)* SYN: Wolfsbane, monkshood, Jacob's chariot, friar's cap FOLK LORE: "Even a man who's pure at heart and says his prayers at night can become a werewolf when the wolfsbane blooms, and the moon is full and bright."	Whole plant — Crude extract	Alkaloids (0.2 to 1.5%) consisting of aconitine, picraconitine, aconine, and napelline. Also aconitic acid, itaconic acid, succinic acid, malonic acid, fructose, melibiose, mannitol, starch & resin.	No longer in use. The British used a tincture of aconite in 1914 to make liniment (mixed with belladonna), but this can be absorbed into the skin & cause poisoning.	A fast-acting poison. As little as 2 mg. is fatal. (The bane of wolves may be used to ward off werewolves.)	Belladonna (deadly nightshade)	Due to toxic nature, no percents are given.

Herb name, synonyms, folk use	Parts used — Extracts	Typical substances	Cosmetic use	Properties and other uses	Similar plants	Comments
ADDER'S TONGUE (*Erythronium americanum*) SYN: Serpent's tongue, dog's tooth, yellow snowdrop	Leaves & bulbs — Glycolic	Constituents of plant have not been analyzed.	Used as a poultice and applied to swellings.	Emollient and antiscrofulous properties; an emetic.	Plants in the lily family.	Used as a soothing and healing agent at 1:1 extract to water.
AGAR-AGAR (*Gelidium amansii*) SYN: Japanese isinglass	The dried mucilage after boiling seaweed. Mucilage is dried to powder form.	Not fully determined. Free amino acids, sugars, and polysaccharides.	Used as emulsion, suspending agent, and gel. Gives a smooth, soft feel.	Hydrophilic— used in fruit, meat, fish as gel filler or gel binder. Maximum level of use is 0.4%.	Other algaes: *agal, gigartina speciosa, euchema spinolum, algin.*	Thickener and gel. Use according to product.
AGRIMONY (*Agrimonia eupatoria*) SYN: Church steeples, cockleburr, sticklewort	Entire plant — Glycolic, essential oil	Volatile oil obtained by distillation, tannin 5%.	Its ability to contract tissue is used for large pores & skin eruptions, acne, and oily skin.	Astringent, tonic, diuretic, eye wash, yellow dye, wound healer, and gargle.	Peruvian bark, hemp, agrimony, water, boneset, eupatorium, gravel root.	Fluid extract 10 to 60 drops as needed in cosmetic formula.

Herb name, synonyms, folk use	Parts used — Extracts	Typical substances	Cosmetic use	Properties and other uses	Similar plants	Com- ments
ALFALFA (*Leguminosae*) FOLK MEDICINE: As a nutrient to increase vitality and weight.	Aerial parts — Crude and extract	Saponins (2 to 3%), soya- sapogenols, vitamins A, B, C, D and E. Triacontanol (which is a plant growth regulator and increases the growth of corn, rice, and bar- ley), flavones, enzymes, calci- um, amino acids.	Used in peel- able face masks. Reported use in treating skin conditions including radiotherapy.	Antifungal properties, estrogenic activities, cholesterol low- ering proper- ties. Used as cattle feed and sprouts for health food enthusiasts.		Alfalfa can be taken as a tea. The leaves are rich in vitamins and minerals.

Herb name, synonyms, folk use	Parts used — Extracts	Typical substances	Cosmetic use	Properties and other uses	Similar plants	Comments
ALOE VERA (*Aloe barbadensis*) SYN: Bitter aloe, cape aloe, cape, curacao aloe FOLK MEDICINE: Used as a stimulant and an antispasmodic; in Chinese medicine to treat headaches. When fresh gel is squeezed from the leaf, it relieves burns & sunburns. It is a skin moisturizer.	The gel inside the leaf. The farmers in the mountains of South America take the entire felet-like gel from the leaf in one piece. This makes an excellent "rub-on" skin treatment and moisturizer. I use this type of "felet" instead of the processed liquid aloe. — Glycolic extract, aloe fluid, aloe dry extrat.	Contains carthartic anthraglycosides (barbaloin), a glucoside of aloeemodin. 4.5 to 25% aloin. Aloe also contains glucomannan, a polysaccharide similar to guar & locust bean gums. Galactose, xylose, and ararinose, steroids, enzymes, amino acids, "biogenic stimulators," saponins, wound healing hormones.	Celltherapy creams, moisturizers, sun screens, refreshing lotions, and tonics.	Emollient, demulcent, sunscreen, food. Maximum levels of about 0.02% in alcohol (186 ppm) and non-alcohol (190 ppm) in laxative.	*Refreshers:* camomile, mallow, linden. *Dehydrated skin:* coneflower, horsetail, St. John's wort, walnut. *Sun screen:* St. John's wort, walnut, PABA, willow bark, titanium-dioxide, African butter, jojoba oil, Cuttlefish oil.	Aloeemodin like buckhorn has been said to have anticancer activity (J.M. Kupchan, A. Karim, Lloydia, 39, 223, 1976). Sometimes guar and locust bean gum is mixed with aloe vera to increase its glucomannan and viscosity. Fresh leaf extract can be used to ensure quality.

Herb name, synonyms, folk use	Parts used — Extracts	Typical substances	Cosmetic use	Properties and other uses	Similar plants	Comments
ALLSPICE *(Pimenta officinalis)* SYN: Pimento, Jamaica pepper, British pimento water (British pharmacopoeia): Oil of pimento: 1 fl/oz Alcohol 12 fl/oz Distilled water 20 fl/oz (Deleted—Talc: 1 oz)	Fruit & shell — Essential oil oleoresin, berry and leaf oils. Allspice N.F. Official F.C.C.	Major component is pimento or eugenol (60 to 80%); methyleugenol, cineole, caryophyllene, protein, lipids, carbohydrates, vitamins A, B_1 (thiamine), B_2 (riboflavin), B_3 (niacin), C & minerals.	Fragrance oil (spicy & exotic odor). Used in islands as after shave and splash.	Aromatic, antiperiodic. Used in alcoholic beverages, dairy desserts, candy, baked goods, etc. Highest food use is 0.025%.	Carolina allspice or sweet bush *(calycanthis floridus)*	Aromatic carminative at dose of 0.05 to 0.2 ml.

Herb name, synonyms, folk use	Parts used — Extracts	Typical substances	Cosmetic use	Properties and other uses	Similar plants	Comments
ALMONDS SWEET— *Amygdalus communis, var. dulcis* BITTER— *Amygdalus communis, var. amara* FOLK MEDICINE: In Chinese medicine, kernels of apricot, peach, and almonds contain tumor treatment. This is known today as the anticancer drug Laetrile.	Kernels — Essential oil	Both oils contain 35 to 55% fixed oil. In bitter almond oil, there's 3-40% amygdalin, but only trace or none at all in sweet oil. Protein (18-20%), emulsin, prunasin, daucosterol, sterols, zinc, calcium oxalate, copper, and tocopherols. Fatty acids: palmitic, stearic, lauric, myristic, oleic, and linoleic.	Excellent emollient for chapped hands (sweet); used in lotions and creams.	Essential oil emollient.	Apricot kernels (*P. armeniaca*)	Sweet almond oil is used in doses of up to 30 ml as laxative. Oil is used in lotions, creams, and ointment bases.

Herb name, synonyms, folk use	Parts used — Extracts	Typical substances	Cosmetic use	Properties and other uses	Similar plants	Com-ments
ALTHEA ROOT (*Althaea officinalis*) SYN: Marshmallow root, mallards, mauls, schloss tea FOLK MEDICINE: Used for over 2,000 years in Europe both internally and externally as a wound healer, for coughs, sore throats, stomach troubles, and in ointments for dry or chapped skin.	Leaves, root, and flowers — Crude extracts	The mucilaginous polysaccharides form 6.2 to 11.6% and are composed of L-thamnose, D-galactose, D-galacturonic acid. Contains sugar, fats, tannin, asparagine, calcium oxalate, pectin.	Used in moisturizing and astringent formulas as a soothing agent. In hand and body creams.	Emollient, demulcent. Used in some foods at very low level of 0.002% (20 ppm).	Other plants of mallow family	In France the tops and leaves are eaten as a spring salad for their property in stimulating the kidneys.

193

Herb name, synonyms, folk use	Parts used — Extracts	Typical substances	Cosmetic use	Properties and other uses	Similar plants	Comments
AMBRETTE SEED (*Abelmoschus moschatus*) SYN: Musk seed, musk mallow FOLK MEDICINE: Used as stimulant and antispasmodic; Chinese medicine for headaches.	Seed (oil) — Essential oil	The floral musk odor is due to ambrettolide and (2)-5-tetradecen-14-olide. Also contains phospholipids, palmitic and myristic acids.	Gives pleasant non-animal musk fragrance to sophisticated perfumes, soaps, creams, and lotions. Use level is 0.12%.	Aromatic, antispasmodic	Musk type plants	A musk for those who don't like the animal musk oil. This herb is also a good astringent having the effect of contracting the tissues. One ounce of the herb can be added to a pint of boiling water and used as a gargle or as a wash for skin ulcers and sores. A good gargle for throat and mouth.

Herb name, synonyms, folk use	Parts used — Extracts	Typical substances	Cosmetic use	Properties and other uses	Similar plants	Comments
ANGELICA (*Archangelica officinalis*) SYN: Garden angelica, European angelica FOLK MEDICINE: The Chinese have used ten angelica species to make "dang-gui," a drug for female ailments for thousands of years.	Roots, leaves, seeds — Crude extracts and oil. Root and seed oil are N.F., U.S.P. and F.C.C.	Contains 0.3 to 1% volatile oil: linolool, bornpol, acetaldehyde, anselicin, osthfenol, archangelicin, etc. Also resins, starch, plant acids, essential fatty acids, sugars.	Has soothing effect on nerves of the skin when applied topically. Has fragrance use.	Diaphoretic and expectorant. Bergapten & xanthotoxin, etc., like bergamot oil, can be phototoxic. (The seed oil is not phototoxic.) Also exhibits antibacterial and antifungal properties.	Bergamot	The bergapten, xanthotoxin and the other coumarins have been shown to be effective in treating psoriasis. One ounce of the powdered root of this herb can be added to a pint of boiling water as a tea for coughs and shortness of breath. Root women use this herb to treat wounds and sores on the body when other methods have failed.

Herb name, synonyms, folk use	Parts used — Extracts	Typical substances	Cosmetic use	Properties and other uses	Similar plants	Comments
ANNATTO (*Bixa orellana*) SYN: Arnotta, annotta, achiote, and achiotillo	Dried pulp of fruit — Crude oil and water soluble extracts	Contains bixin and norbixin, which are carotenoids but have no vitamin A activity.	Used as color	Used as annatto color for foods in about 0.25% maximum.	Carrot oil	Can lose color strength with storage.
APRICOT OIL (*Prunus armeniaca*)	Kernels (oil) — Essential oil	Apricot kernels yield 40 to 50% fixed oil similar to almond and peach kernel oil. Contains olein, glyceride of linoleic acid. Also amygdalin used in Laetrile cancer treatment.	Has softening action on the skin. Used in soaps, lotions, creams, and fragrances. The ground kernels have been used to make face scrubs and facial masks.	Essential oil emollient	Almond oil	I have used apricot oil in skin care products with great success. I have used the ground kernels and seeds in facial masks. Laetrile is the well known and controversial cancer treatment.

Herb name, synonyms, folk use	Parts used — Extracts	Typical substances	Cosmetic use	Properties and other uses	Similar plants	Comments
ARAROBA (GOA) (*Andira araroba*) SYN: Goa, chrysarobin, bahia powder, Brazil powder, vouchapoua araroba	Medullary substance of stems and branches — Powder	Contains several substances but owes its power to chrysophanol-anthranol. Contains quinone and chrysophanic acid which is also found in buckhorn berries (*Rumox eckolianus*).	Astringent, skin treatment (Goa can stain clothing yellow or brown, but the stains can be removed with benzene).	Herbal treatment for acne, eczema, and psoriasis. It is a gastrointestinal irritant.	Cabbage tree (*Andira inermis*)	In India and South America, goa has been esteemed for the treatment of psoriasis, ringworm, and itching. The action of Goa on the skin is not germicidal; it has a chemical affinity for the keratin elements of the skin. I have used goa in a face moisturizer for oily-type skin and in an amino acid gel for acne with great results.

Herb name, synonyms, folk use	Parts used — Extracts	Typical substances	Cosmetic use	Properties and other uses	Similar plants	Comments
ARISTOLOCHIA (*Aristolochia clematitis*) SYN: Birthwort, Dutchman's pipe.	Green parts and root — Glycolic	Main constituent is aristolochine. It has never been carefully analyzed.	Can be used in amounts up to 20% in skin care creams for skin regeneration (celltherapy).	Anti-inflammatory, anti-paralytic, antiperiodic, aphrodiasic.	Snakewort, aloe, echinacea	Aristolochia is a well-tried medicinal with wound-healing, granulating, and epithelizing effects.
ARNICA (*Arnica montana*) SYN: Mountain tobacco, leopard's bane FOLK MEDICINE: Has been used as a diaphoretic, diuretic, stimulant, and vulnerary.	Roots & flowers — Glycolic essential oil	Contains up to 1% of a viscous volatile oil composed of fatty acids: palmitic, linoleic, myristic, and linolenic acid; vitamins A, B, C, and D; triterpenic alcohols, phytosterols, carotenoids, & flavonoids.	Flower extract is used for hair tonics, lotions, creams, massage lotions for cellulitis. Also for perfumes and topical treatments for bruises and sprains.	Essential oil stimulant, coadjutant in the treatment of cellulitis. Limited food use.	*Similar stimulant extracts:* ginseng, nettle, rosemary, sage. *Similar coadjutants for cellulitis:* birch, ivy, horse chestnut, bladderwrack.	Arnica is also used in deodorants along with calendula extract and vitamin E to reduce body odor. Do not use over 0.5% in cosmetic formulas.

Herb name, synonyms, folk use	Parts used — Extracts	Typical substances	Cosmetic use	Properties and other uses	Similar plants	Comments
AVOCADO (*Persea americana*) SYN: Alligator pear, avocato, ahuacate FOLK MEDICINE: The pulp has been used as a hair pomade to stimulate hair growth; used for wounds, as an aphrodisiac, and emmenagogue. Indians used the seeds for dysentery and diarrhea.	Pulp oil (avocado oil) and seed oil — Glycolic essential oil	Pulp oil consists mainly of glycerides of oleic acid, sterols, amino acids, and vitamin D (more than in milk). Mexican avocado leaves contain 3.1% of an essential oil that is 95% estragole and 5% anethole.	The pulp oil is used as a massage oil, in creams, lotions, and hair products. The seed oil has been patented for use in treatment of sclerosis of the skin. Pulp is used in face creams.	The essential oil and the pulp has been used for thousands of years as food; a good source of vitamin D and potassium.		A condensed flavanol isolated from avocado seeds has been reported to have anti-tumor activity against Sarcoma 180 and Walker 256. This flavanol is known as 4,8 Biscatechin (M. DeOliveira, An. Acad. Brasil Cienc., *Chem. Abstr.*, 75, 1973). I have used the oil and the pulp of avocados with excellent results in face creams and facial masks.

Herb name, synonyms, folk use	Parts used — Extracts	Typical substances	Cosmetic use	Properties and other uses	Similar plants	Comments
BALM OF GILEAD (*Commiphora opobalsamum*) SYN: Popular buds and balsam poplar buds FOLK MEDICINE: Used for minor aches and pains; for colds and coughs; topically on sores, cuts, and bruises.	Resinous juice of the bark. — Glycolic liquid (juice); oil obtained is about 1/10 the amount of juice.	Contains 2% volatile oil, resins, salicin, populin; phenolic acids, chalcones, and others.	Topical use for cuts, sores, and bruises. Little use in cosmetics though balsams are used in hair conditioners (i.e., balsam of tolu).	Stimulant, expectorant, anti-pyretic, anti-rheumatic, analgesic.	Balsam Peru, balsam tolu.	Major use of this herbal extract is in cough syrups with white pine, wild cherry bark, bloodroot, and spikenard root. Salicin (the glucoside or salicyl alcohol) is medicinal.

Herb name, synonyms, folk use	Parts used — Extracts	Typical substances	Cosmetic use	Properties and other uses	Similar plants	Comments
BALSAM OF PERU *(Myroxylon perairae)* SYN: Tolufera pereira FOLK MEDICINE: Reportedly used in treating cancer (J. L. Hartwell, *Lloydia*, 33, 97; 1970).	Oleoresinous liquid — Glycolic liquid	Contains 50 to 60% high-boiling volatile oil called cinnamein and 20 to 28% resin which is mainly benzoic and cinnamic acid esters (traces of styrene, vanillin, coumarin).	In perfumes (maximum 0.8%); also in soaps, creams, and lotions.	Antiseptic, aromatic oil	Balsam tolu	In recent years, balsam Peru and balsam tolu are in hair conditioners.
BALSAM TOLU *(Myrospermum toluiferum)* SYN: Balsam tolutanum FOLK MEDICINE: Reportedly used in treating cancer (see above).	Oleoresinous liquid — Glycolic liquid	Contains cinnamic and benzoic acids and volatile oils composed of these acids and their esters with small amounts of terpenes.	In hair conditioners, soaps, creams, lotions, and perfumes (maximum 0.1% in soaps and 0.2% in perfumes).	Antiseptic. A few people may be allergic to balsam tolu. Used in cough medicines, lozenges, etc. Used to compound benzoin tincture.	Balsam Peru	Balsam tolu is most popular in hair conditioners for its fragrance and mild antiseptic qualities.

Herb name, synonyms, folk use	Parts used — Extracts	Typical substances	Cosmetic use	Properties and other uses	Similar plants	Comments
BASIL, SWEET (*Ocymum oasilum*) SYN: Basil FOLK MEDICINE: Used for head colds and as a cure for warts. Widely used as a medicinal herb in China and India (Basil comes from the Greek *basileus*—king— because of its royal fragrance.)	Herb — Essential oil oleoresin	The volatile oil contains d-linalool, methyl chavicol; also protein (14%), carbohydrates (61%) and high concentrations of vitamins A and C.	Fragrance ingredient in perfumes, soaps, and hair products.	Antiwormal activity. Used as a spice and in chartreuse liqueur. Oleoresin used in major food products in low levels of .005% or lower. Can be used as insect repellent on the skin.	Basil rush, wild basil	The basil plant is sacred to both Krishna and Vishnu and is held in high esteem in every house in India. Every good Hindu goes to rest with a basil leaf on his breast. This is his passport to the Elysian fields.

Herb name, synonyms, folk use	Parts used — Extracts	Typical substances	Cosmetic use	Properties and other uses	Similar plants	Comments
BEARSFOOT (*Polymnia uvedalia*) SYN: Uvedalia, leaf cup, yellow leaf cup	Root — Essential oil (fluid extract)	Complete analysis is not known, but probably contains fatty acids, some quinone and maybe chrysophanic acid.	Known as a treatment for hair loss and is used in many hair ointments and lotions.	Anodyne, laxative, and stimulant. It is valued for the treatment of malaria.		To use as a hair tonic, formulate with an herbal alcohol or witch hazel. To use as a hair growth lotion, mix with jojoba oil or lanolin.
BEET JUICE, RED (*Beta vulgaris, Chenopodiaceae*) SYN: Spinach beet, sea beet, garden beet, mangel wurzel	Root — Juice	Betalains (quaternary ammonium amino acids) are the coloring agents in red beet juice. High in glucoses and fine sugars. A treacle principle in the glucose renders it even more nutritious.	Used to a limited extent as a color in cosmetics.	Used to color foods to a limited extent. Used as a food and health juice. In Russia, used to make borsch.		The red color is stable at pH 4.5 to 5.5, but outside this range the color is altered, due to the destruction of betalain at about pH 3.3.

Herb name, synonyms, folk use	Parts used — Extracts	Typical substances	Cosmetic use	Properties and other uses	Similar plants	Comments
BEESWAX (*Apis mellifera*) SYN: White beeswax, yellow beeswax FOLK MEDICINE: In Chinese medicine, beeswax is dissolved in hot wine and taken as a treatment for diarrhea, hiccups, and pain.	Wax obtained from honeycombs Resin from bark — Resin oleoresin tincture	Yellow and white beeswax contains 71% fatty acid esters. One substance in the wax, myricyl alcohol, has been shown to be a plant growth stimulator, and has increased yields of tomato, cucumber, and lettuce.	Thickener, emulsifier, stiffening agent in ointments, cold creams, lotions lipsticks, etc. Also used to remove hair by beauty salons.	Also used in foods as thickener, emulsifier, and flavor ingredients (use levels are low; the maximum is 0.05%).	Jojoba wax	White beeswax is obtained by bleaching yellow beeswax with peroxides. It is on the FDA GRAS (generally recognized as safe) list, but some people are allergic to beeswax.
BENZOIN (*Styrax benzoin*) SYN: Benzoin gum, gum benjamin, Siam benzoin, Sumatra benzoin		Chiefly contains cinnamic and benzoic acid esters. Sumatra benzoin has 70 to 80% of these acid esters and 12% free benzoic acid.	Can be used as an astringent and antiseptic. Benzoin tincture is used as a skin protectant and styptic on small cuts. Also as a preservative.	Antioxidant, preservative, astringent. Certified as natural food flavor. Use level is low maximum 0.014%.		Chief product is benzoic acid used as sodium benzoate in beverages. Tincture of benzoin (B.P. and U.S.P.) is .50 to 1 drachm.

Herb name, synonyms, folk use	Parts used — Extracts	Typical substances	Cosmetic use	Properties and other uses	Similar plants	Comments
BERGAMOT (*Monarda didyma*) SYN: Scarlet monarda, oswego tea, bee balm	Herb — Essential oil	Thymol is the main substance, though this oil is also obtained from *Monarda puctata*.	Fragrance used in soaps, lotions, creams, and perfumes.	Oswego tea is made from the leaves.	Mint, horse-mint, similar also to berg-amot orange oil	The whole plant has the "bergamot orange" fra-grance.
BERGAMOT OIL (*Citrus bergamia*)	Peel of fruit — Oil taken from peel	Three hundred compounds are present in the peel oil from this fruit.	Extensively used in perfumes and eau de cologne. Also in creams and lotions. Used 0.25% in cosmetics and 3% in perfumes.	Due to the pres-ence of bergap-ten it is photo-toxic. Effective in the treatment of psoriasis.	Mint, horse-mint, similar also to berg-amot orange oil.	Though this oil is on the FDA's GRAS list for use in food as a flavor, there are allergic reactions to it.
BETULLA (*Betula pendula*) SYN: White birch, bouleau, berke, bereza	Leaves and bark — Birch glycolic extract	The essential oil contains tannis, a triterpenic pentacyclic der-ivative (*betulin*) and saponins high in methyl salicylate (98%).	Used in sham-poos, lotions for greasy hair, astringent lot-ions, creams for oily skin, body massage lotions for cellulite.	Astringent, mild skin purifier, coadjutant in treatment of cel-lulitis. Anti-inflammatory, anti-pyretic, analgesic.	*Astringents:* witch hazel, rhatany *Skin purifiers:* rosemary, sage *For cellulite:* ivy, horse chestnut, bladderwrack	

Herb name, synonyms, folk use	Parts used — Extracts	Typical substances	Cosmetic use	Properties and other uses	Similar plants	Comments
BISTORT (*Polygonum bistorta*) SYN: Osterick, snakeweed, Easter mangiant, adderwort, twice writhen	Root extract	Never been carefully analyzed. Contains 20% tannin, starch, gallic acid, and gum.	One of the strongest astringents, but is not used in cosmetics though it would be superior to alcohol and acetone.	Astringent, styptic	Witch hazel, rhatany, betulla	The European white birch (*Betula pendula roth*) is used for psoriasis, eczema and other skin problems.
BLADDER-WRACK (*Fucus vesiculosis*) SYN: Fucus, seawrack, kelpware, quercia marina	Thallus — Glycolic extract (0.1% iodine) and fluid extract	Alginates, iodine, mineral salts, sugars, amino acids, fucosterol.	Can be used in foam baths, gels, massage lotions for cellulite. It also has soothing properties when applied to the skin.	Soothing, coadjutant in external treatment of cellulitis. It is also a valuable natural fertilizer.	Other seaweeds have similar properties. Laminaria digitata is an excellent moisturizer. Also kelp.	In 1862 bladderwrack was found to be a good weight reducer. A "cod liver oil" known as Fucol is obtained by roasting bladderwrack with a bland vegetable oil.

Herb name, synonyms, folk use	Parts used — Extracts	Typical substances	Cosmetic use	Properties and other uses	Similar plants	Comments
BOIS DE ROSE OIL (*Aniba rosaeodora*) SYN: Rosewood oil, cayenne rosewood oil	Bark — Glycolic extract from wood	Major component is linalool (90-97%), cayenne bois de rose oil, Brazilian oil.	Used in perfumes, soaps, creams, lotions, in max. amounts of 1.2%.	Used in some foods in max. amounts of 0.003% (24.9 ppm).	Plants with linalool.	
BONESET (*Eupatorium perfoliatum*) SYN: eupatorium, feverwort, thoroughwort, agueweed FOLK MEDICINE: Tonic, febrifuge, diaphoretic, emetic, and for skin rashes.	Herb — Crude extracts, but not readily available	Contains flavonoids, terpenoids, triterpenes, sterols and resins.	Little or no commercial use in cosmetics, but is used by herbalists for skin problems.	Stimulant, febrifuge, laxative, diaphoretic.		One of the effects of this herb is to produce perspiration, and it is therefore called a diaphoretic. I consider it an excellent remedy for catarrh or serious coughing fits. It can be taken hot for coughs and cold as a tonic. Mix an ounce to a pint of water.

Herb name, synonyms, folk use	Parts used — Extracts	Typical substances	Cosmetic use	Properties and other uses	Similar plants	Comments
BORONIA ABSO-LUTE *(Boronia megastigma)*	Flower — Essential oil	Contains ionones, and eugenol.	Used in expensive perfumes.	Aromatic, flavor for fruit type flavors.		The ionones are reported to be allergenic.
BRYONY *(Tamus communis)* SYN: Black bryony, blackeye root, bryonia	Root — Crude extract	Never been analyzed.		Cathartic. Can be poison if taken internally.	European bryony and white bryony	Freckles: When the root powder is mixed with water and applied as a paste it removes freckles.
BUCKTHORN, ALDER *(Rhamnus frangula)* SYN: Frangula, buckthorn, arrow wood. FOLK MEDICINE: Used in cancer treatment as a component of Hoxsey cancer cure.	Bark — Crude extracts	Contains 3 to 7% anthraquinone glycosides, tannis, flavonoids, and anthra-quinones.	Extract is reported to be useful in sunscreen products.	Tonic, laxative, cathartic	Common buckthorn, sea buckthorn, others	A fluid extract of the bark is an excellent laxative and far milder than the commonly used cascara sagrada which has taken its place.

Herb name, synonyms, folk use	Parts used — Extracts	Typical substances	Cosmetic use	Properties and other uses	Similar plants	Comments
BUTCHER'S BROOM (*Ruscus aculatus*) SYN: Kneeholly, knee holly, kneeholm, Jew's myrtle FOLK MEDICINE: It was recommended by Dioscorides and other ancient physicians as a diuretic.	Rhizome — Glycolic extract	Essential oil resins, saponins (1.8% saponosides).	For delicate and sensitive skin.	Diaphoretic, diuretic, skin-lightener, anti-redness, astringent	Similar astringents: birch, escin, witch hazel, rhatany Similar sedatives and lighteners: marigold, camomile horse chestnut, linden tree	

Herb name, synonyms, folk use	Parts used — Extracts	Typical substances	Cosmetic use	Properties and other uses	Similar plants	Comments
CAJEPUT OIL (*Melaleuca leucadendron*) SYN: Cajuput, punk tree, paper bark tree. FOLK MEDICINE: Used for various skin problems.	Leaves & twigs — Essential oil	Contains 14 to 65% cineole, pinene, phenone (10%), terpineol, nerolidol, and traces benzaldehyde and valeraldehyde.	Used as fragrance component in soaps, creams, lotions, and perfumes (Max. 0.4% in perfumes).	Carminative, stimulant, diaphoretic, antimicrobial, and antiseptic.		
CALAMUS (*Acorus calamus*) SYN: Sweet flag, sweet root, sweet cinnamon, sweet myrtle, sweet sedge FOLK MEDICINE: Used for over 2,000 years in China to treat arthritis, strokes, and skin diseases.	Root — Essential oil	Contains asarone, asarylaldehyde, calamene, linalool, calamol, calameone, eugenol, methyl eugenol, azulene, pinene, cineole, camphor, etc.	Used mainly as a fragrance in soaps, creams, lotions, perfumes (0.4%).	Considered toxic and not approved for food use. May be carcinogenic (D.L. J. Opdyke, Food Cosmet. Toxicol., 15, 623, 1977).	Calamus draco	Should not be confused with Calamine Lotion.

Herb name, synonyms, folk use	Parts used — Extracts	Typical substances	Cosmetic use	Properties and other uses	Similar plants	Com-ments
CALENDULA or MARIGOLD (*Calendula officinalis*) SYN: Caltha officinalis, golds, marygold	Flowers, herb leaves — Glycolic liposoluble extracts	Carotenoids, oleanolic acid, mucilages, essential oil.	Freshening tonics, after-sun products, softening hand creams, and sensitive skin lotions.	Stimulant, demulcent, softener, freshener.	Sedatives: camomile, mallow, linden tree Skin brightener: witch hazel, horse chestnut, butcher's broom	Calendula has recently been used in deodorants.
CAMOMILE or CHAMOMILE German: (*Matricaria chamomilla*) Roman: (*Anthemis nobilis*) SYN: Wild chamomile FOLK MEDICINE: Camomile has been used since ancient times for skin problems, and as hair color.	Flowers, herb — Camomile glycolic extract; camomile liposoluble fluid extract: azulenic essential oil	Camomile contains volatile oil (0.25 to 1.9%); flavonoids (apigenin, apigentrin, apiin, rutin, luteolin); plant acids and fatty acids, a polysaccharide with d-gaiacturonic acid, amino acids, etc. Chamazulene and "blue" chamazulene in some species.	Both camomiles are used in cosmetics including bath oils, hair dyes (for blond hair), shampoos, sun protection creams, face masks, and creams. Camomile has a sedative and emollient effect and acts as a normalizer for rough skin.	Chamazulene, a major component, has pain-relieving, wound-healing, anti-spasmodic, anti-inflammatory, and anti-microbial properties. Three sesquiterpene lactones have been reported to have anti-tumor activities *in vitro* against human tumor cells.	Similar sedatives: marigold, butcher's broom, linden tree Similar emollients: aloe, mallow Similar skin normalizers: cone flower St. John's wort oil	Camomile is used in perfume formulas at up to 0.4%. "Blue" camomile is very rare and high in azulenic content. It has a much different fragrance from the "yellow" variety of camomile. Blue camomile is very expensive, but has a lovely fragrance.

Herb name, synonyms, folk use	Parts used — Extracts	Typical substances	Cosmetic use	Properties and other uses	Similar plants	Comments
CAMPHOR (*Cinnamonum camphor*) SYN: Laurel camphor, gum camphor.	Gum from tree — Oil of camphor	The chief constituent of the oil is borneene.	Tiny amounts can be used in after shave lotions or shaving creams. Also in antiseptic and cooling creams.	Antiseptic, stimulant, anti-inflammatory.	Menthol and eucalyptus	Useful in cleansing creams and to relieve the irritation and itching of the sexual organs due to yeast infections (combined with menthol and eucalyptus).
CANANGA OIL (*Cananga odorata*)	Flowers — Essential oil	Contains B-caryophyllene, benzyl acetate, benzyl alcohol, farnesol, borneol, methyl salicylate, benzaldehyde, safrole, linalool, eugenol, etc. (over 100 compounds).	Used as a fragrance in soaps, creams, lotions, and perfumes. It is popular in men's fragrances. Used at a max. level of 0.8% in perfumes.	Essential oil. Also used as a flavor in foods.	Ylang-ylang oil (*canangium odoratum*)	

Herb name, synonyms, folk use	Parts used — Extracts	Typical substances	Cosmetic use	Properties and other uses	Similar plants	Comments
CARAWAY *(Carum carvil)* SYN: Caraway seed, caraway fruit, and carium. FOLK MEDICINE: Used as an anti-spasmodic, carminative, expectorant, and stomachic; also to relieve menstrual discomfort.	Fruit or leaves — Caraway oil N.F.	Contains 4 to 7% volatile oil, 15% lipids, 20% protein, mannan, and flavonoids.	The oil is used in toothpaste, mouthwash, soaps, creams, lotions, and in perfumes (0.4%).	Essential oil, antispasmodic, stomachic, carminative. Used in foods, especially baked goods.		In Shake-speare's *Henry IV*, Squire Shallow invites Falstaff to a hot roasted dish of caraways. The custom of serv-ing a saucerful of caraway with roasted apples is still kept up at Trinity College, Cambridge, and at some of the old London livery dinners just as in Shakespeare's day.

Herb name, synonyms, folk use	Parts used — Extracts	Typical substances	Cosmetic use	Properties and other uses	Similar plants	Comments
CARDAMON (*Elettaria cardamomum*) SYN: Amomum cardamomum; Alpinia cardamomum; cardamon seeds	Dried ripe seeds — Essential oil	Up to 10% volatile oil, 10% protein, 10% fixed oil, 20 to 40% starch, manganese and iron.	Used as fragrance in soaps, creams, lotions, and shampoos. Used at a max. level of 0.4% in perfumes.	Carminative, stimulant	Locust bean gum and other types of seaweeds.	In China the species *Amomum cardamomum* is used in herbal medicine.
CARRAGEENAN (*Chondrus crispus*) SYN: Carrageen, chondrus, carrahan, and Irish moss. FOLK MEDICINE: Considered as a demulcent and a nutrient. Also used for coughs, bronchitis and intestinal problems.	Dried plant — Powdered extract	Carrageenan is a sulfated straight-chain galactan of d-galactose and 3,G-anhydro-D-galactose. It contains a gelling fraction (K-carrageenan) and a nongelling fraction.	It is used in cosmetics as a binding agent, emulsifier, and stabilizer. It is used as such in toothpaste, hand lotions, and creams.	Anti-coagulant, hypotensive, immuno-suppressive. Used in foods extensively.		Some carrageenan is believed to be toxic though the food grade is considered safe. Tests have shown that carrageenan lowers blood cholesterol.

Herb name, synonyms, folk use	Parts used — Extracts	Typical substances	Cosmetic use	Properties and other uses	Similar plants	Comments
CARROT OIL (*Daucus carota*) SYN: Carrot, wild carrot, and Queen Anne's lace. FOLK MEDICINE: Used in China to treat chronic dysentery and as an anthelmintic.	Dried fruit and root — Glycolic: seed oil or root oil	Contains carotol, daucol, limonene, B-bisabolene, B-elemene, geraniol, geranyl acetate, B-carotene and vitamin A (as well as other substances).	Though used primarily as a fragrance and coloring agent in cosmetics, it is very useful in sunscreens as a source of B-carotene and vitamin A.	Soothing, diuretic, emmenagogue. Used as a food color.		Carrot oil used in skin lotions exhibits usefulness for dry as well as oily skin. Also useful in anti-acne skin treatments.
CASSIE ABSOLUTE (*Acadia farnesiana*) SYN: Sweet acacia, husiache, and popinac.	Flowers — Essential oil	25% volatile oil composed mainly of benzyl alcohol, methyl salicylate, geraniol, and over 40 other compounds.	This absolute is used in high-cost perfumes; also used in bath oils for dry skin.	Anti-spasmodic, aphrodisiac, food flavoring.		Root has supposedly been used in Venzuela to treat stomach cancer (J.L. Hartwell, Lloydia, 33, 97, 1970).

Herb name, synonyms, folk use	Parts used — Extracts	Typical substances	Cosmetic use	Properties and other uses	Similar plants	Comments
CASTOR OIL *(Ricinus communis)* SYN: Rincinus palma christi, castor bean, and castor seed oil. FOLK MEDICINE: Castor oil has been used since ancient times in India, Egypt, and China as a carthartic.	Seeds — Oil	Contains mostly triglycerides of ricinoleic acid (90%); other fatty acids are linoleic, oleic, stearic, and di-hydroxy-stearic acids.	Used in lipsticks, hair grooms, ointments, creams, and lotions.	Cathartic, anti-sticking agent, solvent. Used in candy as hardening and anti-sticking agent.		The main objection to castor oil is its nauseating taste and the sickness often produced after its use. Its largest use is industrial.

Herb name, synonyms, folk use	Parts used — Extracts	Typical substances	Cosmetic use	Properties and other uses	Similar plants	Com- ments
CATECHU (Black & Pale) (*Catechu nigrum & uncaria gam- bier*) FOLK MEDICINE: Both types of cat- echu have been used to stop nose- bleeding, also for treating sores and ulcers; reported use in treating cancer (J.L. Hartwell, Lloydia, 33, 97, 1970).	Heartwood, leaves & twigs — Essential oil	Black catechu contains 2 to 20% 1- and dl- catechin; up to 50% cate- chutannic acid. Pale catechu contains 30 to 35% d- and dl- catechin and catechutannic acid (24%).	Both types are used as astrin- gents.	Astringent, anti- bacterial. Tannic acid is consid- ered toxic.		

Herb name, synonyms, folk use	Parts used — Extracts	Typical substances	Cosmetic use	Properties and other uses	Similar plants	Comments
CEDARWOOD OIL (*Thuja occidentalis*) SYN: Cedar oil, white cedar, thuja oil FOLK MEDICINE: Used as ointment or decoction to treat arthritis, coughs, fever, and skin rash.	Leaves, twigs, & wood — Essential oil	Contains thujone, isothujone, l-fenchone, borneol, 1-bornyl acetate, dl-limonene, camphor, myrcene, terines, etc.	Usually used as fragrance ingredient in soaps, shampoos, creams, lotions, bath oils, and perfumes.	Expectorant, stimulant, and counter-irritant.	Other wood oils (pine wood, etc.)	Due to its high thujone content, the oil is poisonous in large quantities. Has been used in treating condyloma and cancers (J. L. Hartwell, Lloydia, 33, 288, 1970).
CENTAURY (*Cantaurium arythraea*) SYN: European centaury, bitter herb, feverwort FOLK MEDICINE: Used as a stomachic and 250 sedative.	Herb leaves — Glycolic	Bitter glucosides, alkaloids, phenolic acids, fatty acids, and triterpenes.	Due to its soothing and astringent properties, it is useful in skin care products. Used in lotions to remove freckles, spots, and skin blemishes.	Bitter tonic, sedative, antipyretic.	Canchalagua (Centaury herb of Chile)	This herb was used in ancient Egypt to treat hypertension and for kidney stones. J. L. Hartwell reported in Lloydia (1969) that it has been used to treat cancers.

Herb name, synonyms, folk use	Parts used — Extracts	Typical substances	Cosmetic use	Properties and other uses	Similar plants	Com-ments
CHAULMOOGRA (*Taraktogenos kunzii*) SYN: Chaulmugra, chaulmogra FOLK MEDICINE: Has been used internally and externally for skin diseases, scrofula, arthritis, eczema, bruises, sprains, and wounds.	Oil of seeds — Oil	Contains chaul-moogric acid, palmitic acid, glycerol, phy-tosterol, and fatty acids.	Used in oint-ments, lotions, and creams for the treatment of psoriasis and eczema.	Sedative, anti-irritant, healing.	The allied species *Glynocardia odorata* and *hydnocarpus*	When applied topically to pso-riasis, the oil breaks up lesions much the same as goa, but will not stain as does goa. In Great Britain, the fatty oil is known as gynocardia oil; in the U. S., it is known as *oleum chaulmoograe*.
CHICLE (*Manilkara zapota*) SYN: Sapodilla	Latex in the bark, pith, and leaves — Gum	Contains 15 to 20% hydrocar-bons that are polyisoprenes, 55% yellow resin, and a gum composed of xylan.	This is a useful natural gum for hair dressings and hairsprays.	Used in chew-ing gum (20%) with sugar, corn syrup, and fla-vorings.		The trade name Chicklets is based on this tree gum.

Herb name, synonyms, folk use	Parts used — Extracts	Typical substances	Cosmetic use	Properties and other uses	Similar plants	Comments
CHINA (*Smilax china*) SYN: Smilax, China shrub FOLK MEDICINE: Used in China for gout and skin problems.	Herb — Glycolic	Contains steroids, smilagenin, sitosterol, glycosides, and saponins.	Used in herbal medicine for skin disease.	Diaphoretic, tonic. When mixed with alum, a yellow dye is produced; when mixed with sulfate of iron, a brown dye is produced.	Sarsaparilla	This plant should not be confused with the "china" used in homeopathy which is Peruvian bark.
CINCHONA (Red & Yellow) Red: (*Chinchona sucirubra*) Yellow: (*Cinchona calisaya*) SYN: Red bark, Peruvian bark, cincho ruba, fever-bark, China bark. FOLK MEDICINE: Malaria & fevers. Used in China to treat hangovers.	Bark — Glycolic	Contains 16% quinoline alkaloids consisting mainly of quinine, quinidine, cinchonine, and cinchonidine. Also tannins, bitter glycosides, resins, and waxes.	Used in hair tonics to stimulate hair growth and control oiliness. Also in gels for aging and troubled skin.	Stimulant, and anti-malarial. Quinine is obtained from red cinchona and used as a bitter in tonic water.	Other stimulants used for the skin: arnica, ginseng, nettle, rosemary, sage.	

Herb name, synonyms, folk use	Parts used — Extracts	Typical substances	Cosmetic use	Properties and other uses	Similar plants	Comments
CINNAMON (*Cinnamomum zelanicum*) SYN: Ceylon cinnamon, and Saigon cassia.	Bark and leaves — Glycolic	Up to 4% volatile oil, tannins, resins, mucilage, gums, sugars, calcium oxalate (two insecticidal compounds, cinnzelanin and cinnzelanol.)	The oil is used as a fragrance in mouthwash, toothpaste, and gargles.	Antiseptic, carminative, anti-fungal, and as a spice in food.		
CITRONELLA OIL (*Cymbopogon nardus*)	Dried grass — Essential oil	Citronellal, geraniol, citronellol, linalool, monoterpene, hydrocarbons (limonene, pinene, camphene, etc.), phenols, and alcohols.	Used as a fragrance in soaps, hair tonics, disinfectants, and perfumes.	Anti-bacterial, anti-fungal.		Some people are allergic to citronella oil.

Herb name, synonyms, folk use	Parts used — Extracts	Typical substances	Cosmetic use	Properties and other uses	Similar plants	Com- ments
CLOVE OIL (*Suzygium aromaticum*) SYN: Eugenia aromatica	Buds, stems, and leaves — Essential oil	The buds con- tain 1 to 18% volatile oil, the stems only 4 to 6%, and the leaves 2 to 3%. Contains gluco- sides, sterols, and esters.	Used in per- fumes, in denti- frices, creams, and lotions.	Carminative, anti-emetic, counter-irritant.		This oil is, of course, known to reduce the pain of a toothache.

Herb name, synonyms, folk use	Parts used — Extracts	Typical substances	Cosmetic use	Properties and other uses	Similar plants	Comments
COCOA (*Theobroma cacao*) SYN: Theobroma FOLK MEDICINE: Cocoa butter has been used for years to reduce wrinkles and for dry skin.	Seeds — Cocoa powder, butter, and syrup	Contains over 300 volatile compounds, hydrocarbons, monocarbonyls, esters, lactones, proteins (18%), fats (cocoa butter), amines, theobromine (0.5 to 2.7%), etc.	Cocoa butter is used as a suppository, ointment base, emollient, skin softener, and protectant.	Also used as a food flavoring ingredient.		Some people are allergic to cocoa butter.
COLTSFOOT (*Tussilago farfara*) SYN: Horsehoof, ass's foot, foalswort	Leaves, flowers, & roots — Glycolic	Contains phytosterol, tannin, silica, amino acids (cystine), dihydride alcohol, and faradial.	Due to the cystine and silica content of this herb, it is excellent for shampoos and conditioners for damaged hair, and in skin moisturizers.	*Tussilago* means "cough dispeller" and a tobacco is made with coltsfoot to help reduce coughs and sore throat. Also used in cough drops with horehound, marshmallow and ivy.	Horsetail	Coltsfoot is high in cystine and silica—excellent for the hair. A tobacco can be made by combining coltsfoot, buckbean, eyebright, betony, rosemary, thyme, lavender and camomile.

Herb name, synonyms, folk use	Parts used — Extracts	Typical substances	Cosmetic use	Properties and other uses	Similar plants	Comments
COMFREY (*Symphytum officinale*) SYN: Comfrey, knitbone, knit-back, slippery root, boneset. FOLK MEDICINE: Used to treat a wide variety of ailments.	Roots & leaves — Glycolic, and powdered allantoin	Root contains 0.75 to 2.55% allantoin, pyrrolizidines, lithospermic acid, muco-polysaccharides (29%), glucose, fructose, d-glu-coronic acid, tannins, carotenes, glycosides, saponins, etc.	Comfrey root and its extract, allantoin, are used in a wide variety of cosmetics.	Anti-inflamma-tory, astringent, demulcent, emollient, hemostatic, expectorant.		The healing and emollient properties of this herb can be used in many products. The muco-polysaccha-rides and allantoin can be used in celltherapy.

Herb name, synonyms, folk use	Parts used — Extracts	Typical substances	Cosmetic use	Properties and other uses	Similar plants	Comments
CONEFLOWER (*Centaurea cyanus*) SYN: Bluebottle, bluebow, blue cap, bluet. FOLK MEDICINE: This herb was known as a tonic, stimulant, and emmenagogue. Also an active wound healer. The blue juice of the herb was once used as a water color.	Flower — Glycolic	The blue extract of coneflower is cyanin and contains many flavones. Contains 3,5-diglucoside, and gallo-catechin, known for their antiseptic and astringent action. Also various flavonoids and amino acids.	In France an eyewash is made with coneflower water (called *eau de casselunettes*). It is excellent in toners, astringents, and healing or cell-therapy creams.	Used in potpourri to give a lovely blue color.	Blessed thistle	The Latin name of this species refers to the goddess Floral; the name of the genus is derived from the centaur Chiron who taught mankind the healing virtue of herbs. Hence, this is a healing herb.

Herb name, synonyms, folk use	Parts used — Extracts	Typical substances	Cosmetic use	Properties and other uses	Similar plants	Comments
CORN SILK (*Zea mays*) SYN: Stigmata, maydis and zea. FOLK MEDICINE: Used as diuretic in urinary problems. In Chinese medicine it is used to treat diabetes and hypertension.	The long styles and stigmata of the pistils called "corn silk" — Powdered extract	Corn silk contains 2.5% fats, 0.12% volatile oils, 3 to 8% gums, 2.7% resin, 1.5% glucosides, 3.8% saponins, vitamins C and K, etc.	Used in face powders	Diuretic, hypoglycemic. Also used as flavoring in some foods.		
CUCUMBER (*Cucumis sativa*) SYN: Cowcumber	The whole fruit peeled and unpeeled — Crude pulp and juice	Cucumber contains up to 96% water. The seeds are similar to pumpkin seeds.	Used in facial creams, lotions and cleansers.	Astringent, soothing properties.		The juice of a cucumber mixed with glycerine and rosewater in equal parts is excellent for sunburns.

Herb name, synonyms, folk use	Parts used — Extracts	Typical substances	Cosmetic use	Properties and other uses	Similar plants	Comments
ECHINACEA (*Echinacea angustifolia*) SYN: Black sampson, coneflower	Roots — Glycolic essential oil	Large amounts of inulin, inuloid, sucrose, bulose, betaine, phytosterols and fatty acids.	Used in creams and lotions. Used for greasy skin as gel or lotion.	Texturizer, firming agent, coadjutant in treatment of wrinkles.	*For firming:* horsetail, ginseng *Skin texturizing:* camomile, St. John's wort	Used in combination with aristolochia and aloe in celltherapy.
ELDER FLOWERS (*Sambucus nigra*) SYN: Black elder, pipe tree, hylder, hylan tree	Bark, leaves, flowers & berries — Glycolic essential oil	Essential oil composed of fatty acids (66%) and alkanes (7%), sterols, flavonoids, flavone glycosides, phenolic acids, rutin, pectin, etc.	In Europe elder flower water is used for eye and skin lotions. Flower essential oil is used in perfumes.	Diuretic, astringent, laxative, diaphoretic.		Used combined with other herbs in hair and skin products. Known for elderberry wine and elderberry tea.

Herb name, synonyms, folk use	Parts used — Extracts	Typical substances	Cosmetic use	Properties and other uses	Similar plants	Comments
ELECAMPANE (*Inula helenium*) SYN: Elf dock, wild sunflower, scabwort.	Root — Glycolic, essential oil	Contains 1 to 4% volatile oil including alantolactone (elecampane camphor), azulene, inulin, sterols. etc.	Used in soaps, creams, lotions and perfumes.	Diuretic, tonic, diaphoretic, antiseptic, astringent.	Spikenard, samphire	A natural blue dye can be extracted from the root. A distilled water of the leaves is an excellent face wash.
ELM, SLIPPERY (*Ulmus fulua*) SYN: Red elm, moose elm, Indian elm. FOLK MEDICINE: For coughs, colds, sore throats. A pinch of the powdered bark on a tooth kills pain.	The inner bark — Glycolic, mucilage, and powdered bark.	The mucilage in the cells of the bark is similar to that found in linseed. Contains starch, calcium, & gums.	Used as thickener and in creams and ointments.	Demulcent, emollient, nutrient, expectorant, diuretic. Wide use for coughs, bronchitis. The bark will preserve oils from becoming rancid (antioxidant).	*Fremontia california* has similar properties but is not related to slippery elm.	An herbal ointment can be made by combining 3 oz. marshmallow leaves, 2 oz. slippery elm bark powder, 3 oz. jojoba wax or beeswax, 16 oz. jojoba butter or lard.

Herb name, synonyms, folk use	Parts used — Extracts	Typical substances	Cosmetic use	Properties and other uses	Similar plants	Comments
EUCALYPTUS (*Eucalyptus globulus*) SYN: Blue gum tree, stringy bark tree FOLK MEDICINE: Used as antiseptic, febrifuge, and as expectorant in respiratory ailments. Also used for burns, wounds, & ulcers.	Oil of the leaves — Essential oil	Contains 0.5 to 3.5% volatile oil, tannins, polyphenolic acids, flavonoids, wax, aldehydes, etc. 70 to 85% eucalyptol gives it cooling, antiseptic properties.	Used as fragrance in soaps, creams, lotions, and perfumes. Also used in liniments, cleansers, and bath oils for spas. When used in creams it reduces itching of yeast infections.	Antiseptic, expectorant, antibacterial. Used in small amounts in some foods, cough drugs, and eucalyptol candy.	Menthol	This is an excellent oil in skin care and in bath oils, but it must be used in tiny amounts (less than 1.0%). It can be toxic in large amounts, although it is non-irritating and non-photo-toxic to the skin.
EYEBRIGHT (*Euphrasia officinalis*) SYN: Euphrasia	Herb — Fluid extract	The precise constituents are unknown. Contains a tannin called euphrasia-tannin acid, mannite, glucose.	Classically used as an eye lotion and eye wash.	Tonic, astringent, used in British herbal tobaccos for coughs.	Bartsia	1 teaspoon eyebright extract and 1 teaspoon goldenseal make an eye lotion for eye disorders.

Herb name, synonyms, folk use	Parts used — Extracts	Typical substances	Cosmetic use	Properties and other uses	Similar plants	Comments
FENNEL (*Foeniculum vulgare*) SYN: Fenkel, sweet fennel, and finocchio	Seeds, leaves, & roots — Oil extract	Seeds contain 1.5 to 8.6% volatile oil: 9 to 28% fixed oil composed of oleic acid, linoleic acid, and high concentrations of tocopherols, flavonoids, protein (16 to 20%), sugars, vitamins, minerals (calcium and potassium).	Fennel and sweet fennel oil are used as a fragrance in soaps, shampoos, lotions, creams, and perfumes.	Carminative, anti-bacterial, cytotoxic properties; weight loss properties.		The ancient Greeks called this herb *maraino* from *maraino*, to grow thin. The seeds, leaves, and root are used in drinks for weight loss. Milton in *Paradise Lost* says: "Grateful to appetite, more pleased my sense/than smell of sweet fennel."
FENUGREEK (*Trigonella foenum graecum*) SYN: Foenugreek, Greek hay.	Seeds — Liquid and spray-dried form	Contains simple alkaloids, choline, lysine, saponins, flavonoids, tryptophan, vitamins A, B and C.	Used in soaps, creams, lotions, and perfume bases. In Java, it is used as hair growth tonic.	Used in foods and in spices. A good source of sapogenins for the manufacture of steroid hormones.		Fenugreek was introduced in Chinese medicine during the Sung Dynasty (1057 A.D.) for kidney ailments, hernia, impotency.

Herb name, synonyms, folk use	Parts used — Extracts	Typical substances	Cosmetic use	Properties and other uses	Similar plants	Comments
FRANKINCENSE (*Boswellia thurifera*) SYN: Olibanum	Gum from bark — Resin	65% resins, 6% volatile oil, 20% water, soluble gum, bassorin 8% and alibano-resin.	Used as fragrance material in exotic type perfumes.	Stimulant. Principally used for incense.	Balsam (tolu or Peru)	In ancient Egypt, the kohl used to paint the eyelids was made from charred frank-incense.
GERANIUM OIL (*Pelargonium gravedens*) SYN: Algerian geranium oil, bourbon geranium oil	Leaves & stems — Essential oil	High in herbal alcohols such as citronellol, geraniol, linalool, and ketones, aldehydes, menthol, & acids.	Rose geranium oil is widely used as a fragrance component in soaps, creams, lotions, and perfumes.	Anti-fungal and anti-bacterial activities *in vitro*. Some use in foods.		Some people are allergic to geranium oil.

Herb name, synonyms, folk use	Parts used — Extracts	Typical substances	Cosmetic use	Properties and other uses	Similar plants	Comments
GINGER (*Zingiber officinale*) SYN: Common ginger, Nigerian root. FOLK MEDICINE: Used as carminative, diaphoretic, and appetite stimulant. Used for thousands of years in China for many ailments including baldness and arthritis.	Root — Ginger oil, powdered root, and oleoresin	Contains 1 to 3% volatile oil and pungent principals (*gingerols and shogaols*): 6 to 8% lipids (triglycerides, phosphatidic acid, lecithins, fatty acids); protein (9%); starch (50%); vitamins (especially niacin and A); minerals; amino acids; resins; zingerone; etc.	Ginger oil is used as a fragrance material in some cosmetics. Also used in herbal cosmetics such as men's products, bath oils, body rubs.	Numerous pharmacological properties including stimulating the vasomotor and respiratory centers. Lowers serum and hepatic cholesterol. Carminative properties. Antitussive, nonirritating, nonsensitizing, nonphototoxic. Food use.		I have used ginger in bath oils, sports rubs, and other products. It is "warming" and soothing to tired, sore muscles. It also has anti-oxidative activities in foods.

Herb name, synonyms, folk use	Parts used — Extracts	Typical substances	Cosmetic use	Properties and other uses	Similar plants	Comments
GINSENG Oriental ginseng (*Panax ginseng*) American ginseng (*Panax quinquefolius*) SYN: Chinese ginseng, Korean ginseng, seng and sang, man root, man's health. FOLK MEDICINE: Many uses. Oriental ginseng has warming properties, but American ginseng has cooling properties.	Root — Ginseng glycolic extract; ginseng fluid extract (both have 1% saponosides as ginsenoside); ginseng dry extract (has 10% saponosides as ginsenoside)	There are many types and grades of oriental ginseng. It contains many saponins; volatile oil; sterols; starch; sugars; pectin; vitamins (B_1, B_2, B_{12}, nicotinic acid, pantothenic acid, and biotin); choline, fats, minerals (zinc, copper, manganese, calcium, iron, etc.); polyacetylenes; and others.	Used in creams, gels, tonics, and masks; reactivating and wrinkle creams for the skin. Excellent in hair tonics and shampoos.	Stimulant, toner, reactivating agent; reduces stress, and lowers blood sugar. Used as tea and in capsule form.	Plants with similar use for wrinkles: horsetail, coneflower, St. John's wort Plants with similar use as hair stimulant and tonic: arnica, peruvian bark, nettle, rosemary, sage.	Liquid ginseng can be used in hair and skin care products in amounts from 2 to 10%. Powdered ginseng can be used up to 2% in products.

Herb name, synonyms, folk use	Parts used — Extracts	Typical substances	Cosmetic use	Properties and other uses	Similar plants	Comments
GOLDENSEAL (*Hydrastis canadensis*) SYN: Orange root, yellow root, Indian tumeric, eye balm FOLK MEDICINE: Used for hemorrhoids, nasal congestion, sore gums, itchy scalp and dandruff, and acne.	Root — Crude extract (fluid and tincture) and hydrastine salts.	Contains isoquinoline alkaloids (good dandruff treatment); hydrostine (1.5 to 4%); berberine (0.5 to 6%), chlorogenic acid; lipids; saturated and unsaturated fatty acids; resins; sugars; starch.	Limited cosmetic use, but has history as topical for acne, dandruff, & sore eyes.	Anti-convulsive, antiseptic, hemostatic, diuretic, laxative, and tonic. Used as herbal tea.	No plants offer the hydrastis extract but goldenseal.	Berberine, an alkaloid in goldenseal, is similar to hydrastine used in uterine problems and for menstrual pain. Other drug uses. A popular herbal medicine for colds, flu, and viruses is to take a combination of goldenseal and echinacea.

Herb name, synonyms, folk use	Parts used — Extracts	Typical substances	Cosmetic use	Properties and other uses	Similar plants	Comments
GRAPEFRUIT OIL (*Citrus paradisi*) SYN: Shaddock oil, citrus preservative. Recent dermatological studies: grapefruit oil was found non-irritating, non-sensitizing, and non-photo-toxic (D.L.J. Opdyke, *Food Cosmet. Tooxicol.,* 12, 723, 1974).	Peel & seed — Grapefruit oil and naringin extract	The peel oil and seed oil contain monoterpenes; limonene (90%); sesquiterpenes; aldehydes; citronellyl; nootka-tone; ketones; 7-gaptens; 7-methoxy-8-2-formyl-2-methyl-propyl; other substances.	Grapefruit oil from the peel is used as a fragrance in soaps, lotions, creams, and perfumes. Grapefruit seed oil is used as a preservative in cosmetics.	Seed oil has been used for herpes and skin problems in South America and in water to destroy bacteria. Used as a weight reducer in capsules.	Other citrus oils	I have created a preservative using grapefruit seed oil with other natural extracts. Excellent preservative action and non-toxic. The preservative action is due to various esters. This is the best natural preservative I have found. It is known as grapefruit seed extract and citrus seed extract. I combine the extract with vitamins A, C and E.

Herb name, synonyms, folk use	Parts used — Extracts	Typical substances	Cosmetic use	Properties and other uses	Similar plants	Com- ments
GUAR GUM (Cyamopsis tetragonoloba)	Endosperm of seed — Powdered extract for various viscosities	Contains 80% guaran (a galacto-mannan); 5 to 6% protein; 10 to 15% moisture; 2% fiber; 0.5 to 0.8% ash.	Used as a binder and thickener in lotions and creams.	Lowers the serum and liver cholesterol. Used as a thickener and stabilizer in foods. An appetite suppressant.	Gum arabic, gum tragacanth	
GUAIC WOOD OIL (Bulnesia sarmienti) SYN: Champaca wood oil	Root — Oil	Up to 72% guaiol, bulnesol, and guaioxide.	Used as fixative, modifier or fragrance oil in soaps, creams, lotions, and perfumes .	Used as flavor component in foods and beverages. Non-irritating, non-sensitizing, non-phototoxic		

Herb name, synonyms, folk use	Parts used — Extracts	Typical substances	Cosmetic use	Properties and other uses	Similar plants	Comments
HAWTHORN (*Crataegus oxyacantha*) SYN: May, may-blossom, white-horn, ladies' meat, cuckoo's beads	Dried haws or fruit — Glycolic	Amygdalin crataegin, & other constituents.	Cardiac, diuretic, astringent, tonic.	Can be used in creams, lotions, and hair tonics as astringent.	Other plants of the order *Rosaceae*: *Crataegus aronia, C. odoratissima, C. azarole*.	
HEARTSEASE (*Viola tricolor*) SYN: Wild pansy, love-lies-bleeding, love-in-idleness, loving idol.	Herb: leaves, flowers, & seeds — Glycolic	Main constituent is violin (an emeto-cathartic substance), resin, mucilage, sugar, salicylic acid).	A strong decoction of the syrup is recommended for skin problems.	Tonic, expectorant, demulcent, cathartic. Medical journals say it's valuable for a skin disorder called *crusta lactes*, or "scald head."	Violet	Love-in-idle-ness is still used in Warwickshire as a love charm (heart-sease). It was used by Puck in *A Midsummer Night's Dream* as a love charm.

Herb name, synonyms, folk use	Parts used — Extracts	Typical substances	Cosmetic use	Properties and other uses	Similar plants	Comments
HENNA (*Lawsonia alba*) SYN: Henna, Ac-khanna, Egyptian privet, Jamaica mignonette FOLK MEDICINE: Leaves have been used for centuries in Middle East, Far East, and North Africa as dye for nails, hands, hair, cloth-ing, and for treat-ing skin problems, headaches, jaun-dice, etc.	Flowers, leaves, stems, root. (Only leaves have coloring principal). — Crude extract	Contains 0.55 to 1.0% law-sone (2-hy-droxy-1,4 naphtho-quinone), 5-10% gallic acid and tannin, 11% sugars and resin. Lawsone is the active color principal. It is not in the bark, stem, or root—just in the leaves.	Used in hair care products as dye, condi-tioner, and rinse. Dye can turn hair "orange" unless mixed with indigo and oth-er dyes.	Lawsone has anti-fungal (fungicidal and fungistatic) activity against alternaria, aspergilus, absidia, penicil-lium, and other species. Only 0.1% (1000 ppm) is active as fungicide. The gallic acid and 1,4-naph-thoquinone also have anti-bacte-rial activities		Henna is mixed with indigo and logwood to obtain different shades. For long-lasting results, a pH of 5.5 must be obtained (i.e., citric acid added). The non-coloring henna makes an excellent ingredient for shampoos and neutral rinses. When non-col-oring henna is mixed with peppermint it is excellent for oily type hair (in shampoo and hair rinses).

Herb name, synonyms, folk use	Parts used — Extracts	Typical substances	Cosmetic use	Properties and other uses	Similar plants	Comments
HONEYSUCKLE (*Lonicera caprifolium*) SYN: Dutch honeysuckle, goat-leaf (Fr. chevrefeuille).	Flowers, seeds, leaves. — Glycolic (essential oil)	There is little uniformity in composition, and its constituents have not been analyzed.	Used for its fragrance and cleansing properties. A popular soap in France, Le Petit Marseillais, contains honeysuckle. (It's available in the U.S. health food stores as Honeysuckle Vegetal Soap.)	Expectorant, laxative, diuretic, anti-spasmodic, and emitico-cathartic properties	There are 300 species of *Caprifoliaceae*	Culpepper says: "Honeysuckles are cleansing. It is an herb of Mercury and therefore for the lungs. It is a cure for asthma and takes away the evil of the spleen...in an ointment ,it will clear the skin."

Herb name, synonyms, folk use	Parts used — Extracts	Typical substances	Cosmetic use	Properties and other uses	Similar plants	Comments
HOPS *(Humulus lupulus)* SYN: European hops, common hops FOLK MEDICINE: Used for treating diarrhea, insomnia, and nervous conditions.	Flowers — Crude and essential oil	Contains 0.3 to 1.0% volatile oil: 3-12% bitter principals (i.e., humulone, cohumulone, etc.). Glycosides, rutin, phenolic acids, tannins, lipids, estrogen.	Used in skin creams and lotions in Europe for its skin softening properties.	Antimicrobial sedative, estrogenic properties. Used in some foods at maximum levels of 0.072%.		Hops contain phytohormones responsible for toning and calming nervous skin. "A pillow of hops brings calm sleep."
HOREHOUND *(Marrubium vulgare)* SYN: Marrubium, horehound, and white horehound FOLK MEDICINE: An ancient well-known treatment for sore throat, colds, and coughs.	Herb — Crude extract	Contains 0.3 to 1.0% of a bitter called marrubiin (a diterpene lactone): alcohols 0.29% choline: 0.3% betonicine; volatile oil; resin, tannin, wax, fat, sugar.	Little commercial cosmetic use though an ointment with horehound syrup is good for wounds.	Diuretic properties, also a source of natural sweeteners. Expectorant and tonic.	Hyssop (also contains marrubiin)	A simple tea made of horehound is excellent for the common cold.

Herb name, synonyms, folk use	Parts used — Extracts	Typical substances	Cosmetic use	Properties and other uses	Similar plants	Comments
HORSE CHESTNUT (Aesculus hippocastanium) SYN: Ippocastano, robi-castanie.	Seeds — Glycolic extract (with 1% escin)	Escin and other triterpenic saponins, purinic derivatives, amino acids, B vitamins, and flavonoids.	Tonics, lotions for reddened or sensitive skin, protective creams and gel for the hands. Products for cellulitis.	Decongestant, mild astringent, skin lightener, coadjutant in treatment of cellulitis.	Lighteners: marigold Sedative: camomile, butcher's broom, linden tree Cellulitis: birch, ivy, bladder-wrack	
HORSETAIL (Equisetum aruense) SYN: Shave-grass. bottle-brush, pewterwort FOLK MEDICINE: Used to stop bleeding, as external ointment, and internal tea.	Herb — Glycolic	High in silica (silicic acid 7%), starch, sulfur, saponins, malic and oxalic acids, flavonoids, fatty acid esters, amino acids (cystine).	Tonics, lotions, creams to prevent wrinkles, hair products to prevent hair loss and greasy hair.	Texturizer, elasticizer, diuretic, astringent	_For hair:_ coltsfoot _Texturizer and plasticizer:_ coneflower, ginseng _Rough skin & wrinkles:_ marigold, St. John's wort	I have used horsetail combined with coltsfoot and ginseng for the scalp. Scalps that are low in silicic acid, sulfur, and cystine have higher hair loss.

Herb name, synonyms, folk use	Parts used — Extracts	Typical substances	Cosmetic use	Properties and other uses	Similar plants	Com- ments
HYSSOP *(Hyssopus officinalis)* SYN: Common hyssop FOLK MEDICINE: Used in treating sore throat, coughs, and colds.	Herb — Oil	Contains 0.3 to 2% volatile oil, hyssopin (a glucoside), 5 to 8% tannin, fatty acids, hesperidin, diosmin, marrubiin, resin, and gum. Contains over 50 unidentified compounds.	Used externally as a diaphoretic (in baths) and in treating skin irritations, burns, and bruises. Used as a fragrance in soaps, creams, lotions, and perfumes at 0.4% maximum.	Hyssop extracts have been used to treat herpes simplex virus (E.C. Herrmann, J., and L. S. Kucera, *Proc. Soc. Exp. Biol. Med.* 124, 874, 1967). Non-irritating, non-sensitizing, non-phototoxic.	Horehound (also contains marrubiin). Balm oil of lavender.	The fine odor of hyssop essential oil is valued more than oil of lavender. It is also used in a liqueur known as chartreuse. Bee's honey from hyssop is the finest honey!

Herb name, synonyms, folk use	Parts used — Extracts	Typical substances	Cosmetic use	Properties and other uses	Similar plants	Comments
IMMORTELLE (*Helichrysum angustifolium*) SYN: Helichrysum, everlasting FOLK MEDICINE: Use as an expectorant, diuretic, and conditions such as burns, bronchitis, psoriasis, migraine, and allergies .	Flowers and flowering tops — Extracts and oils	Contains 0.075 to 2% volatile phthalides, helipyrone, triterpenes, wax, flavonoids, caffeic acid, nerol, geraniol, linolool, eugenol, and others.	The absolute is used as a fixative and fragrance in perfumes. Extracts are soothing and moisturizing. Can be useful in sun protection products because of UV absorption properties.	Expectorant, antitussive, antiinflammatory, antiallergic agent, UV light absorber, and diuretic. Used for burns, psoriasis, headache, migraine, and allergies.		Immortelle (everlasting) oil has antimicrobial properties *in vitro* against *Staphylococcus aureus*, *Eschenchia coli* and *Candida albicans*.
INDIGO (*Indigofera tinctoria*) SYN: *Pigmentium indicum* FOLK MEDICINE: Used as a natural dye.	Herb — The blue dye is obtained from a yellow chemical known as indocan. On fermentation it turns blue.	Not completely analyzed.	Used as a blue color in cosmetics. It is calming to the scalp.	At one time used as medicine to produce nausea and vomiting but is no longer in use as such.		Indigofera is synthesized and known as indigotine. Often mixed with henna to produce a variety of hair color shades.

Herb name, synonyms, folk use	Parts used — Extracts	Typical substances	Cosmetic use	Properties and other uses	Similar plants	Com- ments
IVY *(Hedera helix)* SYN: Ivy, climbing ivy FOLK MEDICINE: Used as food for cattle. Flowers were used for dysentery and removal of sunburn.	Leaves, berries — Glycolic	Saponins (mainly ederin), chlorogenic, caffeic acids, and flavonoids.	Used in foam baths, creams, and for packs or massage lotions for cellulitis.	Sedative and coadjutant for cellulitis.	Similar sedative plants: marigold, camomile, butcher's broom Similar anticellulitis herbs: birch, horse chestnut, and bladderwrack	

Herb name, synonyms, folk use	Parts used — Extracts	Typical substances	Cosmetic use	Properties and other uses	Similar plants	Comments
JASMINE *(Jasminum officinale)* SYN: Royal jasmine, Italian jasmine, poet's jessamine, and common jasmine. FOLK MEDICINE: In China numerous jasminum species are used for hepatitis, cirrhosis of liver, skin problems, abdominal pain, headaches, and insomnia.	Flower — Essential oil	The aroma of jasmine essence is made up of over 100 compounds. Benzyl acetate is the highest concentration. Also linalool, jasmonates, jasmolactone and jasmonic acid.	The strong aroma of jasmine is widely used in cosmetics and perfumes. Maximum use in perfumes is 0.3%.	In Western culture the essential oil is used as a calmative and as an aphrodisiac.		In China jasmine is known as *Moli* and the Hindus call it "Moonlight of the grove." This yang herb is used in aromatherapy massages. I've used it in many cosmetics and have created a line of hair and skin care products combining jasmine with wild white camellia oil (a traditional Chinese herbal).

Herb name, synonyms, folk use	Parts used — Extracts	Typical substances	Cosmetic use	Properties and other uses	Similar plants	Comments
JUNIPER BERRIES (*Juniperus Communis*) SYN: Genévrier, ginepro, enebro, common juniper berries FOLK MEDICINE: Used as carminative and diuretic. Also to treat colic and gastrointestinal infections. The steam is used for bronchitis.	The ripe, dried fruit and leaves — Essential oil	Berries contain 0.2 to 3.42% volatile oil. Also sugars (glucose and fructose), glucuronic acid, l-ascorbic acid, gallotannins, gei-jerone, and others.	Oil is used in soaps, creams, lotions and perfumes. Also used for skin problems such as acne and eczema. Makes an excellent water for toning the skin.	Diuretic, antiseptic, astringent, and carminative. In foods it is used as a flavor component in gin.		This yang herb, like jasmine, has many uses. The product known as cade oil or juniper tar oil is used in France for chronic eczema.
KARAYA GUM (*Sterculia urens*) SYN: Sterculia gum. Indian tragacanth, kadaya	Dried exudation from trunk of tree — Powder of various particle sizes	Contains a polysaccharide with a high molecular weight (9,500,000 m). It has not been completely analyzed.	Used as a thickener and suspending agent in lotions, creams, and hair-setting products.	Used in foods as binder and to prevent ice crystals in sherberts, ice creams, etc.	Other gums such as gum arabic, gum tragacanth	Karaya gum is able to swell in cold water up to 100 times its original volume.

Herb name, synonyms, folk use	Parts used — Extracts	Typical substances	Cosmetic use	Properties and other uses	Similar plants	Comments
KELP (*Fucus vesiculosus*) SYN: Seaweed, bladderwrack, fucus, and sea-wrack	Entire plant — Glycolic	Alginates, iodine in organic combination with mineral salts, sugars, amino acids, and vitamins A, C, B-complex, & E.	Used in foam baths, creams, gels, and massage lotions for cellulitis.	Due to its high iodine content kelp is used for obesity and to normalize the thyroid.	There are various seaweeds used in cosmetics today (see *bladder-wrack*).	The soothing properties of kelp are similar to aloe and mallow.
LABDANUM (*Cistis ladaniferus*) SYN: Ambreine, rockrose, gum cistus, ciste, and cyste. FOLK MEDICINE: Used as an expectorant and for diarrhea.	Leaves and twigs — Oleoresin and oil	Labdanum gum contains volatile oil, paraffins, and resins. The oil contains over 120 compounds.	Oil is used as fixative in soaps, creams, lotions, and perfumes.	Also used as flavoring in foods.		

Herb name, synonyms, folk use	Parts used — Extracts	Typical substances	Cosmetic use	Properties and other uses	Similar plants	Com-ments
LAVENDER (*Lavandula angustifolia*) SYN: True lavender and garden lavender FOLK MEDICINE: Used internally and externally for many ailments, headache, sprains, acne, sores, and toothache.	Flowering tops — Essential oil (lavender and lavandin)	Contains 0.5 to 1.5% volatile oil, tannin, coumarins, flavonoids, triterpenoids, etc.	Lavender oil is used in antiseptic ointments, creams, and lotions. It is a widely used fragrance material.	Analgesic, anti-convulsive, anti-spasmodic, carminative, sedative, tonic, and stomachic.	Other yang oils are jasmine and juniper berries.	This yang oil is non-toxic, non-irritating, and is not phototoxic. It is used in aromatherapy.
LEMON OIL (*Citrus limon*) SYN: Lemon oil, cedro oil	Rind, juice, oil of peel or seed — Oil	Contains 90% monoterpenes (mainly limonene, sabinene, pinene, and myrene).	Used as a fragrance in soap, creams, lotions, and perfumes.	Used in pharmaceuticals as a flavoring, and in foods. The waxes have antioxidant properties.	Other citrus oils (orange, lime, grapefruit and bergamot).	The seed oils of citrus (especially grapefruit seed) have antioxidant and antibacterial properties.

Herb name, synonyms, folk use	Parts used — Extracts	Typical substances	Cosmetic use	Properties and other uses	Similar plants	Com- ments
LEMON GRASS (*Cymbopogon citratus*) SYN: West Indian lemongrass, Madagascar lemongrass, cochin lemongrass, etc. FOLK MEDICINE: Used in Chinese medicine to treat colds, headache, stomach ache, and rheumatic pain.	Leaves — Essential oil	Contains volatile oil (0.2 to 0.4%), an unknown alkaloid, saponins, hexacosanol, and others. Fragrance comes from citral (65 to 85%), citronellic, linalool, geraniol, etc.	Used as a fragrance component in soaps, creams, lotions, and perfumes.	Anti-microbial, analgesic, anti-pyretic, and anti-oxidant properties. Non-irritating, non-sensitizing, non-toxic.		Lemongrass is used as a starting material for the synthesis of vitamin A.

Herb name, synonyms, folk use	Parts used — Extracts	Typical substances	Cosmetic use	Properties and other uses	Similar plants	Comments
LICORICE ROOT (*Glycyrrhiza glabra*) SYN: Italian licorice, Turkish licorice, glycyrrhiza, and sweet wood.	Dried runners and roots — Crude extracts	The major active principal is glycyrahizinic acid (1 to 2%). Also flavonoids, isoflavonoids, licoflavonol, licoricone, glycyrol, amines, gums, wax, and many aromatic chemicals.	Used only as an aromatic in cosmetics, but can be used as an anti-inflammatory in lotions and creams. Has been sucessful with contact dermatitis.	Estrogenic activities, anti-ulcer, mineralocorticoid, anti-inflammatory, anti-allergic, inhibition of tumor growth (I. F. Shavarev, Vop. Izuch, Ispolz. Soludki, SSR, *Akad Nauk USSR* 167, 1966).		Licorice root is used in traditional Chinese herbal medicine. Glycyrahizinic acid has recently been used as an alternate treatment for the immune system in persons with AIDS.
LITMUS (*Roccella tinctoria*) SYN: Lacmus, orchella weed, dyer's weed.	The whole plant for its pigment. — Liquid	Contains resins, wax, starches, gum, tartrate and oxalate of lime, chlorine, and the color principals are acids or acid anhydrides.	Could be used for color but is not used at present.	Used to make litmus papers for measuring pH.		Used to make blue and red litmus paper.

Herb name, synonyms, folk use	Parts used — Extracts	Typical substances	Cosmetic use	Properties and other uses	Similar plants	Comments
LOCUST BEAN GUM (*Ceratonia siliqua*) SYN: Carob bean gum, carob gum, locust gum	The seeds of carob — Powdered extract	Similar to guar gum with a different d-galactose chain.	See *guar gum*.	See *guar gum*.	Guar gum	Guar gum and locust bean gum are often used together.
LILY-OF-THE-VALLEY (*Convallaria magalis*) SYN: May lily, convallaria, our lady's tears, ladder-to-heaven, Jacob's ladder	Flowers, leaves, whole herb — Essential oil	Contains two glucosides (convallamarin & convallarin), volatile oil, tannin, salts, etc.	Can be used as aromatic material in cosmetics but to get a strong fragrance, many infusions are needed.	Cardiac tonic and diuretic. Action of drug.		The crystalline powder of the active principals acts upon the heart like digitalin.
LIME OIL (*Citrus aurantifolia*)	Whole crushed fruit or juice of the fruit, peel, and seeds. — Distilled lime oil	Contains d-limonene, pinenes, camphene, citral, linalool, bergapten, berga-mottin, and others.	Lime oil is used as a fragrance and fixative in soaps, creams, lotions, and perfumes (up to 1.5%).	Non-irritating, non-sensitizing, and non- phototoxic to human skin.	Other citrus	Lime oil is a refreshing fragrance and can be used in cosmetics. It has a cooling action on the skin.

Herb name, synonyms, folk use	Parts used — Extracts	Typical substances	Cosmetic use	Properties and other uses	Similar plants	Comments
LINDEN TREE (*Tilia cordata*) SYN: Tiglio, linden	Flowers — Glycolic	Essential oil with major constituent being farnesol. Also flavonoids, gallic and catechnic tannins.	Eye tonics, after-sun lotions, emollient lotions for sensitive skin, foam baths, feminine hygiene products.	Refreshener and sedative.	Similar refresheners: aloes, camomile, marigold, and mallow	Up to 5% linden can be used in hair and skin care products.
LOVAGE (*Levisticum officinale*) SYN: Old English lovage, smellage, smallage, and maggi herb. FOLK MEDICINE: Used as a diuretic, stomachic, expectorant, and for skin problems.	Roots, leaves, seeds, stems — Essential oil	Contains from 0.5 to 1.0% volatile oil, angelic acid, resins, (a coloring principal called ligulin), phthalides, glucoside, gum, and resin.	Used as a fragrance component in soaps, creams, lotions, and perfumes (maximum 0.2%).	Used as a flavor component in foods and beverages. Non-irritating, non-sensitizing.	Angelica	I have used lovage to test the purity of water. A drop of lovage oil in pure water will turn to a fine crimson red, but if the water is not pure, the red changes to blue.

Herb name, synonyms, folk use	Parts used — Extracts	Typical substances	Cosmetic use	Properties and other uses	Similar plants	Comments
LUPINS (Lupinus albus) SYN: Lupin, wolfs>bohne FOLK MEDICINE: Used as a diuretic and emmenagogue.	Seeds and herb — Crude extract	Contains a glucoside called lupinin, a crystalline (magolan), dextrin, lupanine, others.	Used in soaps, creams, lotions, and as an external treatment of ulcers.	Anthelmintic, diuretic, emmenagogue.		In 1917 a lupin banquet was given: the table had a lupin tablecloth; lupin beefsteak roasted in lupin oil, lupin bread, lupin cheese, and lupin coffee were served; hands were washed with lupin soap.
MAGNOLIA (Magnolia acuminata) SYN: Cucumber tree, blue magnolia, swamp sassafras FOLK MEDICINE: Used for rheumatism, malaria, and as a laxative.	Leaves and flowers — Glycolic	Contains a crystalline principal magnolin, bitter glucosides, and others.	Used as a fragrance material in soap, lotions, creams, and perfumes.	Mild diaphoretic, tonic, and aromatic stimulant.		It is said that if the bark is chewed it cures the desire for tobacco.

Herb name, synonyms, folk use	Parts used — Extracts	Typical substances	Cosmetic use	Properties and other uses	Similar plants	Comments
MALLOW, BLUE (*Malva sylvestris*) SYN: Common mallow, mauls. FOLK MEDICINE: Used for coughs, colds, for urinary organs.	Leaves and flowers — Glycolic	Flavonoids, anthocyanines, chlorogenic, galacturonic acid, tannins, starch, mucilage, pectin oil, asparagin, cellulose.	Tonics, lotions, emollient lotions and creams, bath products, mouth washes.	Softener, smoother, and emollient	Marsh mallow, musk mallow, sea tree mallow, other mallows (also see *althea root*).	I have used marsh mallow for astringents, and blue mallow as a skin ointment. A "clay mask" of mallow is a skin softening mask.
MINTS: **PEPPERMINT** (*Mentha piperita*) **SPEARMINT** (*Mentha viriois*) **CORNMINT** (*Mentha arvensis*) **PENNYROYAL** (*Mentha pulegium*) FOLK MEDICINE: Peppermint, spearmint, and their oils are used as stomachics, anti-spasmodics,	Herb — Essential oil	Peppermint yields 0.1 to 1.0% volatile oil composed mainly of menthol, menthone, and menthyl acetate. Spearmint yields about 0.7% volatile oil consisting of carvone, dihydrocarvone, phellandrene,	The mints are used mostly as flavoring and fragrances in cosmetics, e.g., flavoring for mouthwashes and lip gloss and fragrance for soaps, rinses, shampoos, rinses, creams, lotions, and perfumes. Spearmint and cornmint have a	Mints are used in foods. Spearmint oil is popular in chewing gum (about 0.132%), and peppermint is popular in candy (about 0.104%). Menthol is extracted from cornmint by freezing, which reduces the amount of	Other mints: marsh mint (*mentha sativa*) wild water mint (*mentha aquatica*) curled mint (*mentha acrispa*) bergamot mint (*mentha citrata*) Egyptian round-leaf mint (*mentha rotundifucia*)	I have used the various mints in many unconventional cosmetics, e.g., in mint hair rinses which are cooling and antiseptic; in unique bath oils with ginger and eucalyptus; in a non-hardening clay mask with sea extracts.

Herb name, synonyms, folk use	Parts used — Extracts	Typical substances	Cosmetic use	Properties and other uses	Similar plants	Comments
and for nausea, sore throat, colds, headaches, toothaches, and cramps. The Japanese menthol plant and Chinese peppermint oil have high quantities of menthol. The Japanese have used menthol for over 200 years and even carried it with them in a tiny silver box. Rats dislike peppermint: in ancient times, rags soaked with peppermint oil were stuffed into rat holes.		limonene, menthone, menthol, and piperitenone. Cornmint yields 1 to 2% volatile oil with a high concentration of menthol (70 to 95%), menthone, menthyl acetate, isomethone, thujione, and piperitone. Pennyroyal yields about 1% of a volatile oil known as pulegiom with a ketone of pulegone.	maximum use of 0.4% and 0.8% respectively as fragrance materials.	menthol from 90% to 55%. Good results with menthol have been obtained for colds, sore throats, and coughs. Menthol is strong and should be used in small amounts (5.967 ppm or less). Pliny the Elder has written about the power of pennyroyal to drive away fleas, and the herb's Latin name (pulegiom) refers to the Latin word for flea—pulex.	horse mint (mentha sylvestrias)	The mints are stimulants, antiseptics, anesthetics, as well as cooling and soothing. Men's shaving and skin care products can make good use of the mints. My most successful skin cleansers and astringents utilize the mints. They have an excellent tonic effect on the skin and seem to work on all skin types.

Herb name, synonyms, folk use	Parts used — Extracts	Typical substances	Cosmetic use	Properties and other uses	Similar plants	Com-ments
MUSK SEED (*Hibiscus aoelmuschus*) SYN.: Ambretta, Egyptian alcee, bamia moschata. FOLK MEDICINE: The Arabians mix the seeds with coffee for their strong, exotic, aromatic flavor. Seeds are also said to be an aphrodisiac.	Seeds — Essential oil	The seeds of this evergreen shrub contain a fixed oil, a col-ored resin, and albuminous matter.	Used for its albuminous extract to make "skin milk" used for dry itchy skin. It can be used to create a vege-tarian musk oil fragrance.	Anti-spasmodic, stomachic, nervine, and as a breath sweet-ener.		

Herb name, synonyms, folk use	Parts used — Extracts	Typical substances	Cosmetic use	Properties and other uses	Similar plants	Comments
MYRRH (*Commiphora myrrha*) SYN: Balsamodendron, myrrha, mosmol, mirna, didthin, bowl FOLK MEDICINE: Used as stimulant, antiseptic, expectorant, antispasmodic, emmenagogue and stomachic.	The oleo-resin from the stem — Crude extract	Contains 1.5 to 17% volatile oil composed of herrabolene, limonene, dipentene pinene, eugenol, comic, resins, cholesterol, and 60% gum.	Myrrh is an excellent astringent and can also be used in mouthwashes and gargles. Also as a fragrance in soaps, creams, lotions, and perfumes (0.8%).	Used as a flavor in foods and beverages. It also has antimicrobial activities, is non-sensitizing, non-irritating, and non-phototoxic.		I have used myrrh for many years in hair and skin care products.
NETTLE (*Urtica urens*) SYN: Common nettle, stinging nettle	Herb, seeds — Glycolic	Contains formic acid, mineral salts, carbonic acid. Also phytosterols (scalp treatment), amino acids, protein, vitamins.	Used in hair and skin products. Said to stimulate hair growth if juice is applied to scalp. Used in hair tonics, skin creams, and astringents.	As a medicinal food, it is high in phosphates and trace minerals such as iron. Nettle juice is a recognized homeopathic tonic.	Plants with similar hair tonic effect: arnica, ginseng, rosemary, sage, Peruvian bark.	I have used nettle in hair tonics, skin astringents, and even to make a "beautiful green color" for cosmetics and colognes.

Herb name, synonyms, folk use	Parts used — Extracts	Typical substances	Cosmetic use	Properties and other uses	Similar plants	Comments
OATS (*Avena sativa*) SYN: Common oats, white oats, panicle oats, groats	Seeds — Powdered extract	Starch, gluten, albumin, protein, sugar, gum oil, and salts.	Popular as a facial mask, used in soaps, lotions, and creams for its cleansing action.	Nervine, stimulant, and antispasmodic.		Herbalists suggest boiling oats in vinegar and applying the mash to "age spots" and freckles.
OLIBANUM (*Boswellia carteri*) SYN: Frankincense and olibanum gum. FOLK MEDICINE: Used since antiquity as incense in India, China, Egypt, and the Catholic church. Called Frankincense. Used in ancient Egypt to make embalming oil for their dead.	Oleogum, from bark of tree — Crude extract as olibanum oil	Contains 3 to 10% volatile oil with 20% gum, and 5 to 8% bassorin. High content of boswellic acid.	It is used as fixative or fragrance in soaps, lotions, creams, and perfumes (0.8%).	This herb has a strong analgesic effect. It has an antioxidative effect on fats and oils, and is therefore a natural replacement for BHA.		

Herb name, synonyms, folk use	Parts used — Extracts	Typical substances	Cosmetic use	Properties and other uses	Similar plants	Comments
OLIVE OIL (*Olea Europea*) SYN: Olea, olea lancifolia, olea oleaster, olivier FOLK MEDICINE: One of the oldest trees is the olive tree. The branch means peace. It was used in the diet and burned in the sacred temples.	Oil of fruit, leaves, bark — Oil	The gum-resin contains benzoic acid and olivile. Mannite is found in the leaves. Also the palmitin, triolein, archidic esters, oleic acid, and other fatty acids.	Olive oil soap is made by mixing olive oil with salt. Warm olive oil is believed to be good for the scalp. Also used in shampoos, conditioners, and moisturizers.	Leaves are astringent and antiseptic. Bark and leaves have febrifugal qualities. The oil is a demulcent and a laxative.	Cottonseed oil, rape oil, sesame oil, and poppyseed oil are often used as adulterants.	Olive oil mixed with witch hazel is a good hair tonic for dry, dull hair. It also relieves stings and burns.

Herb name, synonyms, folk use	Parts used — Extracts	Typical substances	Cosmetic use	Properties and other uses	Similar plants	Comments
ORANGE OIL **Bitter** (*Citrus vulgaris*) **Sweet** (*Citrus aurantium*) SYN: Citrus oil, bitter orange, Seville orange, sweet orange. FOLK MEDICINE: Used as carminative in treating dyspepsia.	Fruit, flowers, peel — Oils are U.S.P. and N.F	Bitter peel contains 1 to 2.5% volatile oil, naringin, rhoifolin, lonicerin, hesperidin, and other flavonoids, rutin, vitamins A, B, C, carotenoid, pectin, citrantin, etc. Sweet peel contains 1.5 to 2% volatile oil, many of the above substances, and vitamin E.	Neroli and petitgrain oils are used as fragrance materials in soaps, creams, lotions, and perfumes.	Anti-inflammatory, antibacterial, antifungal, antihypercholesterolemic.	As antibacterials, similar plant extracts include grapefruit oil, lemon oil, pine needle oil and lime oil.	I have used citrus seed extracts in cosmetics for their preservative qualities for almost twenty years with good results. (Also see *grapefruit oil*.)

Herb name, synonyms, folk use	Parts used — Extracts	Typical substances	Cosmetic use	Properties and other uses	Similar plants	Comments
PAPAIN (*Carica papaya*) SYN: Vegetable pepsin	Latex from unripe fruit — Various grades of powdered extract	Papain is similar to bromelain and ficin, but as an enzyme, it contains no carbohydrates. Contains 212 amino acids, organic salts, furmaric acid, malic acid, di-hydroxyfurmaric acid, and others.	Used in some face creams and cleansers as a "face lift" and skin softener. At one time was used for wounds, sores, ulcers, and psoriasis (topical).	Widely used as meat tenderizer (sometimes combined with bromelain or ficin). Also used in beer to hydrolyze proteins.	Bromelain, ficin	Chymopapain is being studied for use in the treatment of lower back pain.
PARIS HERB (*Paris quadrifolia*) SYN: Herba Paris, true love, one berry	Entire plant — Glycolic	Contains a glucoside called paradin.	A cooling ointment is made from the seeds and juice for skin problems and inflammations.	Poison and narcotic. Should be used internally with caution as overdose is fatal. Tiny amounts have been used for bronchitis, coughs, colic, heart problems.	Other species: *Paris polyphylla*	The seeds and berries have a similar effect to opium. In Russia, the leaves are used for the mentally ill. It's also used as an antidote to mercury andarsenic.

Herb name, synonyms, folk use	Parts used — Extracts	Typical substances	Cosmetic use	Properties and other uses	Similar plants	Comments
PARSLEY (*Petroselinum crispum*) SYN: Garden parsley and common parsley FOLK MEDICINE: Used to treat jaundice, menstrual problems, asthma, coughs, indigestion, gallstones (as tea) and eaten as breath freshener (garnish).	Roots, seeds — Flakes, oil, oleoresin	Contains 2 to 7% volatile oil and 22% fixed oil high in petroselinic acid (octadecenoic acid) and palmitic, myristic, stearic, oleic, linoleic, myristolic acids. Also proteins, vitamins A and C, and sugars. Also furocoumarins and myristicin.	Used as a fragrance component in soaps, creams, lotions, and perfumes (0.2% maximum).	Highly nutritious with pharmacological properties: laxative, hypotensive, antimicrobial and tonic. Contains some furocoumarins which are phototoxic.	Coriander (known as Chinese parsley)	A chemical in parsley, myristicin, is believed to be a psychedelic. Parsley is used as a garnish on top of foods, and is often more nutritious than the foods it garnishes. After a garlic-laden meal, parsley acts as a breath freshener.

Herb name, synonyms, folk use	Parts used — Extracts	Typical substances	Cosmetic use	Properties and other uses	Similar plants	Comments
PATCHOULY OIL (*Pogostemon cablin*) SYN: Patchouli oil FOLK MEDICINE: In Chinese medicine, patchouly is used for colds, headaches, nausea, and stomach pain.	Dried leaves — Essential oil	Contains 1.5 to 4% volatile oil composed mainly of patchouli alcohol, norpatchulenol (both give the oil its odor), cinnamaldehyde, benaldehyde, eugenol, etc.	Extensively used as a fragrance component and as a fixative. Also used for bad breath in mouthwash.	Used as a food flavor. Used for insecticidal activity against insects in stored grains. Antimicrobial and bactericidal properties.		
PECTIN	Obtained from the cell walls of plants, the peel of citrus and apple pomace — Various grades of powder extract. Some are N.F.	Pectin contains dextrose, sodium citrate, potassium carbonates, lactates, and other sugars and salts.	Used as a thickener and film-forming agent in beauty masks. Also in creams and lotions as a thickener and combined with kaolin.	Largest use is in jams, jellies, and preserves.	Other gums: algin, guar, etc.	Pectin has cholesterol-lowering properties and is not digested.

Herb name, synonyms, folk use	Parts used — Extracts	Typical substances	Cosmetic use	Properties and other uses	Similar plants	Comments
PINE BARK, WHITE (*Pinus strobus*) SYN: Eastern white pine FOLK MEDICINE: Used for centuries by American Indians for coughs, colds, congestion, and as a poultice to treat wounds.	Bark — White pine bark extract	Mucilage coniferin, coniferyl alcohol, diterpenoids, volatile oil, and others.	Other pines are used as fragrance materials in cosmetics. Some such as white pine are used in rubs and turpentine linaments. Pine tars are used in bath oils.	Used in some cough syrups.	Various pine species	There are more than 33 species of pines that have medicinal properties.
PINE NEEDLE OIL (*Pinus sylvestrus*) SYN: Swiss mountain pine	Needles — Oil, N.F.	Contains monoterpene; hydrocarbons (d-limonene, camphene, murcene, etc.): sesquiterpenes, alcohols, etc.	Dwarf, Scotch, and Siberian pine oils are used as a fragrance in soaps, creams, lotions, and perfumes (maximum 1-2%). Popular in bath oils.	Antimicrobial, antiviral, antibacterial, nonphototoxic.	Various pine needles	Siberian pine needle extract has the most pleasant fragrance.

Herb name, synonyms, folk use	Parts used — Extracts	Typical substances	Cosmetic use	Properties and other uses	Similar plants	Comments
PIPSISSEWA *(Chimaphila umbellata)* SYN: Pyrola umbellata, wintergreen, king's cure, love-in-winter, rheumatism weed, ground holly FOLK MEDICINE: Used as tea for bladder-stones, externally for sores and blisters. Used for diabetes, diminishes lithic acid in urine, and as replacement for uva-ursi herb.	Dried leaves — Crude extract	Main ingredient is arbutin gum and other glycosides, flavonoids, ursolic acid, methyl salicylate, resins, tannins, gums, starch, sugar, etc.	When the bruised leaves are applied to the skin, they act as a vesicant and rubefacient, which is very efficacious for skin problems.	Astringent, diuretic, antiseptic action on urine, tonic, bacteriostatic properties. Used in some foods.	Pyrola, wintergreen	

Herb name, synonyms, folk use	Parts used — Extracts	Typical substances	Cosmetic use	Properties and other uses	Similar plants	Comments
PRIMROSE OIL, EVENING (*Enothera odorata*) SYN: Tree primrose, evening primrose flowers FOLK MEDICINE: Has been used for dyspepsia, torpor of the liver, and female complaints.	Bark, leaves, seeds — Crude oil	A mixture of essential fatty acids, and one of the best knwon sources of GLA, or gamma-linolenic acid (besides mother's milk).	Recently used in shampoos for dry hair, in lotions and creams for dry skin and eczema, and in hair conditioners.	Astringent, sedative, recently used for premenstrual syndrome and for its GLA content.	Another species, *Enothera biennis*, and a white-flowered species grow in India. Borage oil and black currant seed oil are also high in GLA (gamma-linolic acid).	I first introduced EPO to the U.S. with a line of hair and skin care products. EPO lotion is excellent for eczema and other skin problems. 15 drops of EPO in juice three times a day is excellent for PMS and female problems.
QUILLAIA (*Quillaja saponaria*) SYN: Soapbark, soap tree bark, quillaia, ke-li-ya, murillo bark, panama bark	Dried inner bark — Crude powdered, fluid and saponin extracts	Contains 9-10% triterpenoid saponins consisting of glycosides of quillaic acid tannin; calcium oxalate; sugars; starch; others.	Used in shampoos for its foaming and anti-dandruff properties. Relieves itching and psoriasis scales.	Anti-inflammatory, antimicrobial expectorant; can be toxic if taken in large amounts internally, due to hemolytic and gastrointestinal irritation	Yucca root	I've used quillaia for many years in cosmetics with good results. The powder should not be inhaled during manufacturing, but once in a liquid state, it's nonirritating.

266

Herb name, synonyms, folk use	Parts used — Extracts	Typical substances	Cosmetic use	Properties and other uses	Similar plants	Comments
RHATANY (*Kramena triandra*) SYN: Rhatanhia, mapto, red rhatany	Dried root — Glycolic	Tannins (krameria-tannin), rhatanine (methyl-tyrosine), lignin, gum, starch, mineral acids, others .	Astringent, lotions, and creams. Used in bronzers as suntanning agent.	Astringent, restorer tonic. Used for dysentery, sore throats, and as astringent wash.	Similar for suntanning: aloes, St. John's wort, walnut Astringents: birch, witch hazel	Rhatany glycolic extract is used in amounts from 2 to 10%.
ROSE HIP SEED OIL (*Rosa aff. rubiginosa*) SYN: Rose hips, hip berries, Rosa Mosqueta FOLK MEDICINE: Tea of hips is used for colds, flu, vitamin C. Oil of seeds used for hair, skin, burns, scars.	Hips, and seeds of hips — Ground hips for tea, oil of seeds.	Rose hips contain vitamin C (1.25%), carotenoids, flavonoids, pectin, polyphenols (2.64%), riboflavin, fatty acids.	Hair conditioning creams and shampoos, used in skin moisturizing cream, sun protection creams, healing agent for scars and burns.	The hips are used for a medicinal tea high in vitamin C, anti-inflammatory, anti-scrobutic, moisturizer, mucilaginous.		I first brought rose hip oil to the U.S. from South America and created excellent moisturizers that reduce signs of aging, reduce scars, and burns. Also as shampoo and hair conditioner.

Herb name, synonyms, folk use	Parts used — Extracts	Typical substances	Cosmetic use	Properties and other uses	Similar plants	Comments
ROSEMARY (*Rosemarinus officinalis*) SYN: Polar plant, compass plant, rosmarino FOLK MEDICINE: Herbalists suggest rosemary mixed with borax prevents baldness.	Herb, root — Glycolic extract	About 0.5% volatile oil: flavonoids (diosmetin, hispidulin, etc.); rosmarinic acid; carnosic acid; oleanolic acid; tannins, others.	Widely used in cosmetics as a purifier or toning agent, and as a fragrance material (maximum 1%).	Antimicrobial activities, analgesic activity, nonirritating, and nonsensitizing.	Other skin purifiers: sage Toning agents: arnica, Peruvian bark, ginseng, nettle	I have used rosemary for almost two decades in cosmetics with great success in amounts from 0.5 to 2%. Equal parts of rosemary and sage is an excellent hair rinse.
ROSE OIL (*Rosa alba*) SYN: Bulgarian otto of rose, Bulgarian rose oil, French rose absolute, and rose de mai absolute	Flowers — Rose oil is N.F.; Rosewater is N.F.	Rose oil contains geraniol, citronellol, nerol, B-phenethyl alcohol, geranic acid, and eugenol, which constitutes 55 to 75% of the oil.	Rose oil &rosewater are used as fragrances in soaps, creams, lotions and perfumes (maximum use: 0.2%). Rosewater & glycerine are used together as a skin moisturizer.	Rose oil and absolute are used as flavor ingredients in foods for their fruit-type flavor (use is 2 pm maximum).		In India rosewater is used to make an excellent yogurt drink.

Herb name, synonyms, folk use	Parts used — Extracts	Typical substances	Cosmetic use	Properties and other uses	Similar plants	Comments
RUE *(Ruta graveolens)* SYN: Herb-of-grace, herby-grass, garden rue FOLK MEDICINE: Used as an emmenagogue, antispasmodic, hemostatic, and vermifuge.	Herb — Crude oil is N.F.	Contains a volatile oil (0.1%), rutin (2%), various alkaloids. bergapten, psoralen, and other coumarins.	Rue oil is used as a fragrance in soaps, creams, lotions, and perfumes (0.15% maximum in perfumes). Rue oil is also the source of 2-undecanone, a valuable perfume chemical.	Used as a flavor component in foods (maximum 2 ppm).	Other plants with bergaptens	Since furo-coumarins have phototoxic properties, these extracts can be used to treat psoriasis.
RUTIN SYN: Quercetin-3-rutinoside, rutoside, eldrin.	The glycoside from various species of ferns. — Pure rutin (formerly N.F.)	Can be obtained from eucalyptus leaves, fiola flowers, buckwheat, various ferns.	Can be used in cosmetics for its anti-inflammatory and anti-phototoxic properties.	Main biological activity is the decrease of capillary permeability.		Rutin is nontoxic and has shown the ability to inhibit skin cancer in animals (B.L. Vanduuren, et.al., *J. Natl. Cancer Inst*, 46, 1039, 1971).

Herb name, synonyms, folk use	Parts used — Extracts	Typical substances	Cosmetic use	Properties and other uses	Similar plants	Comments
SAGE (*Salvia officinalis*) SYN: Garden sage, true sage, Balkan sage. FOLK MEDICINE: Is used as a tonic, digestive, antiseptic and astringent.	Leaves — Sage oil	Contains 1.0 to 2.8% volatile oil; picrosalvin, Carnosol, salvin, carnogic acid, flavonoids, camphor, thujone, tannis, others.	Used as a skin purifier and toning agent in shampoos, creams, lotions, gels, masks for greasy skin, wrinkled skin, and as a fragrance component (0.8% maximum).	Phenolic agents in sage give it antimicrobial activity, especially against *staphyloccus aureus*. It's non-irritating, non-sensitizing, nonphototoxic.	Similar skin purifiers: rosemary Toning agents: arnica, Peruvian bark, ginseng, nettle	I have used sage oil for many years in cosmetics with good results from 0.5 to 1.0%. Equal parts of rosemary and sage makes an excellent herbal hair rinse.
ST. JOHN'S WORT (*Hypericum perforatum*) SYN: Iperico, milleportuis, johanniskraut FOLK MEDICINE: Used as aromatic, and for bladder problems, catarrh, and bed-wetting in children.	Herb tops and flowers — St. John's wort oil	Volatile oil (terpenes and sesquitepenes); tannis, flavonoids (hyperin, rutin); hypericin; others.	After-sun oils, creams, lotions, tonics, for reddish or chapped skin, for wrinkles, and as healing agent.	Texturizer, purifier, astringent, soothing agent.	*Other healing agents:* marigold, camomile, coneflower *Astringents:* birch, witch hazel, rhatany *Pre-sun and after-sun:* aloe, walnut, horse chestnut, butcher's broom	I have used St. John's Wort oil in many cosmetics with excellent results (up to 1%). A good quality St. John's wort oil should be a clear, lovely, red color.

Herb name, synonyms, folk use	Parts used — Extracts	Typical substances	Cosmetic use	Properties and other uses	Similar plants	Comments
STORAX (*Liquidambar styraciflua*) SYN: Liquid storax FOLK MEDICINE: Used as an antiseptic and expectorant, and for treating wounds and skin problems.	Balsam of bark — Storax oil is official in U.S.P.	Contains cinnamic acid; styracin; phenylpropyl cinnamate; various styrene; various alcohols (phenylpropyl, benzyl, ethyl); vanillin; others.	Storax oil is used as an ingredient to make benzoic tincture, also as an antiseptic and antimicrobial for preserving cosmetics.	Used in foods, as a flavoring and fixative (0.001%).	Balsam tolu, benzoic gum.	
STRAWBERRY (*Fragaria vesca*) FOLK MEDICINE: Used for dysentery. The once-famous Antioch drink was prepared with stalks to be drunk on the nativity of John the Baptist.	Leaves, fruit — Oil	Cissotanic, malic, citric acids, sugar, mucilage and an unknown aromatic oil (similar to musk, rose, and violet).	The oil of the leaves or fruit can be used for their astringent action in cosmetics.	Laxative, diuretic, astringent		A cut strawberry rubbed over the face immediately after washing will lighten the skin and remove a slight sunburn.

Herb name, synonyms, folk use	Parts used — Extracts	Typical substances	Cosmetic use	Properties and other uses	Similar plants	Comments
SUNFLOWER OIL (*Helianthus annus*) SYN: Marigold of Peru, *sola indianus, chrysanthemum peruvianum* FOLK MEDICINE: Seeds were made into infusion for relief of whooping cough. They have been used in Russia for malarial fever, even where quinine has failed.	Seeds — Sunflower seed oil	Seeds yield 50 to 60% oil. Contains tannis (helianthitanic acid); inulin; levulin; essential fatty acids, others.	Sunflower seed oil is used as an emollient in soap, creams, and lotions. It is a good base for massage oils and lotions.	Diuretic and expectorant properties.		

Herb name, synonyms, folk use	Parts used — Extracts	Typical substances	Cosmetic use	Properties and other uses	Similar plants	Comments
THYME (*Thymus vulgaris*) SYN: Common thyme, garden thyme, and French thyme FOLK MEDICINE: An infusion or tincture of thyme was used for acute bronchitis, laryngitis, coughs, gastritis, and to improve appetite.	Herb — Thymol and thyme oil	Contains 0.8 to 2.6% volatile oil consisting of phenols, monoterpene hydrocarbons, linalool, thujan, thymol, carvacrol, others.	Used in ointments or creams to treat fungal skin infections. Also used in toothpastes, soaps, creams, lotions, and perfumes (0.8%).	Thyme oil has anti-spasmodic, expectorant, and carminative properties; antimicrobial on both bacteria and fungi (due to thymol and carvacrol). Non-irritating, non-sensitizing, and non-phototoxic.	Marjoram, rosemary, sage, oregano, and other plants of mint family have similar anti-oxidative properties	
TRAGACANTH (*Astragalus gummifer*) SYN: Gum tragacanth, gum dragon	Gummy exudation of branches — Flake, powder, ribbon in various grades. Meets U.S.P and N.F. standards.	Consists of 20 to 30% water, soluble fraction of tragacanthic acid and arabinogalactan; acetic acid; bassorin; polysaccharides; others.	Used in creams and lotions as an emulsifier and binding agent; in hairsets as a film-former, and in toothpastes.	Used in foods as an emulsifier and in confectionaries.	Gum arabic	I have used herbal gums for hairsprays and styling gels for years with great results. PVP, a synthetic gum, is easily replaced by these natural gums.

Herb name, synonyms, folk use	Parts used — Extracts	Typical substances	Cosmetic use	Properties and other uses	Similar plants	Comments
VANILLA (*Vanilla planifolia*) SYN: Bourbon vanilla, Reunion vanilla, Tahiti vanilla	Unripe fruit — Crude extract and tincture is N.F.	Contains vanillin and over 150 other aromatic chemicals.	Vanilla extract N.F. is used as a fragrance in soap, lotions, creams, and perfumes.	Used as a flavor in foods and beverages.		
WILD WHITE CAMELLIA (*Camellia oleifera* Abel) SYN: White Camellia, Camellia oil, Mountain Camellia. FOLK MEDICINE: Used in China for hair and skin. As a cancer treatment: camellin extract.	Leaves and seeds — Crude extract (oil) from seeds	Camellia oil is high in essential fatty acids (11%), 75% oleic acid, camellin, camelliagenin A, camellia sapo-genol I, A1-Barrigenol, theasapogenol, hydroxyerythrodiol, vitamins A, B, E, and various minerals: P, Za, Ca, Fe, Mn, Ca, and Mg.	The oil is used as a skin and hair emollient, and has been used in this manner in China and Japan for hundreds of years.	The leaves are used to make green and black tea in China, Japan, and other parts of Asia.		I have made many hair and skin products using wild white camellia oil. I first brought it to the U. S. from the Longevity Village in China. Camellin has been shown to be effective against cancer cells in Chinese studies.

Herb name, synonyms, folk use	Parts used — Extracts	Typical substances	Cosmetic use	Properties and other uses	Similar plants	Comments
WINTERGREEN OIL (*Gaultheria procumbens*) SYN: Checkerberry, teaberry, or gaultheria oil.	Leaf — Oil is U.S.P.	Wintergreen oil contains mainly methyl salicylate (about 98%).	Wintergreen oil is used in body rubs, bath oils, toothpaste, mouthwash.	It has a "heating" and "warming" action on muscles and skin. Tonic, stimulant, astringent, and aromatic.	Sweet birch oil, *betula lenta*, peppermint oil, menthol.	Wintergreen oil used in tiny amounts is great in "sports rub" creams and in "spa bath" formulas.
WITCH HAZEL (*Hamamelis virginiana*) SYN: Hamamelis water, winter bloom FOLK MEDICINE: Used internally to treat mouth and throat irritations, hemorrhoids, eye inflammations, insect bites, burns, and skin irritations.	Bark, leaves — Glycolic extract, hamamelis water	Tannins (Hamamelitannin); essential oil (aldehydes and carboxylic acids); gallic acid; saponins; choline; resins; flavonoids; others	Used as an astringent in creams, lotions, gels, face tonics, aftershaves, fresheners, and masks.	Astringent and hemostatic properties. Witch hazel water is 15% alcohol.	Similar astringents: birch, rhatany Skin lighteners: horse chestnut, butcher's broom	I have used witch hazel in many cosmetics.

Herb name, synonyms, folk use	Parts used — Extracts	Typical substances	Cosmetic use	Properties and other uses	Similar plants	Comments
YARROW (*Achillea millefolium*) SYN: Milfoil, common yarrow, nosebleed, and thousand leaf FOLK MEDICINE: Tonic, carminative, astringent. Used for loss of appetite, stomach cramps, flatulence, gastritis, external bleeding of all kinds, wounds, sores, and skin rashes.	Herb — Crude extract	Contains 0.1 to 1.4% volatile oil which has azulene (51%); pinenes; borneol; cineole; camphor; other compounds. Also flavonoids (rutin); sterols; alkanes; fatty acids and sugars.	Extract can be used in bath oils for soothing effect on the skin, and in creams and lotions	Used in bitters and vermouths, and herb tea mixes. Anti-inflammatory, non-phototoxic.		

Herb name, synonyms, folk use	Parts used — Extracts	Typical substances	Cosmetic use	Properties and other uses	Similar plants	Comments
YLANG-YLANG OIL (*Cananga odorata*)	Flowers — Essential oil	Contains linalool, geraniol, sesquiterpenes, methyl eugenol, hexanoic, and others.	Used as fragrance material in soaps, creams, lotions, and perfumes (maximum is 1%).	Used in foods as flavor component (5.03 ppm). Non-sensitizing, non-phototoxic, non-irritating.		
YUCCA (*Yucca schidigera*)	Leaves — Yucca extract	Contains steroidal saponins. Little else is known of the chemical composition.	Used in shampoos for foaming ability and in soaps.	Hemolytic properties. Non-toxic. Used in foods such as root beer and frothy drinks (618 ppm).	Quillaya bark, sarsaparilla	Yucca root has a great sudsing action as a shampoo. Leaves hair clean and soft.
ZOAPATL (*Montanor tormentosa*) FOLK MEDICINE: Used widely in Mexico as a treatment for menstrual problems.	Leaves — Zoapatl extract	The chemical composition is unknown.	Little is known about cosmetic use, but it is said to have a tonic effect on the skin.	It has alternative, analgesic, anodyne, anti-inflammatory properties.	Devil's claw	Similar to devil's claw in that it can reduce the pain of arthritis.

Chapter 3
The fine art of reading a cosmetics label

At one time, making cosmetics was a craft. Products were natural and were handmade in small batches from herbs.

Today, people spend well over fifteen *billion* dollars a year on cosmetics, and with that kind of money at stake, some companies will use any method they can think of to get you to buy their products. It's a copy-cat business, with manufacturers stealing ideas from each other so rapidly that often the only difference from one label to the next is a new synthetic chemical or a different shade of artificial color.

Cosmetic chemists are an odd group of men (most are men). Lacking in both imagination and concern for humans, animals and the environment, they have no ability to make a product that actually does something for the hair and skin. Instead, they torture lab animals to prove their chemicals are safe (an inaccurate and inhumane form of testing), in collaboration with the agency that's supposed to protect you from them: the Food and Drug Administration (FDA).

Most cosmetic manufacturers will use any kind of slogan to make you disregard their ingredients, which include formaldehyde, benzene and petrochemicals that pollute the environment and don't belong in your hair or on your skin. The FDA's GRAS ("generally recognized as safe") list is designed to protect the chemical industry, not the consumer.

The next four pages compare the back labels of a natural and a synthetic shampoo and a natural and a synthetic moisturizer, followed by my comments on the ingredients (no brand names are mentioned). Following that, I discuss the different sorts of ingredients natural and synthetic manufacturers use. (If you run across any terms you don't know, you can look them up in Chapter 1.)

Since the FDA hasn't seen fit to render you these services, I thought I'd do their job for them.

A natural shampoo label

White Camellia & Jasmine Conditioning Shampoo

Water, Coconut Soap, Vegetable Glycerine, Wheat Protein, Aloe Vera, White Camellia Oil, Rosa Mosqueta® Rose Hip Seed Oil, Macadamia Nut Oil, Almond Oil, Geranium Oil, Lavender Oil, Orange Blossom Oil, Jasmine, French Rose Water, Natural Vitamin E Oil. Preserved with Citrus Seed Extract and Vitamins A, C & E.

Coconut Soap: One of several ways in which this shampoo cleans your hair. When added to wet hair, it combines with your hair's natural oils and rinses away dirt—with extra foaming and cleansing added by the wheat protein. **Vegetable Glycerine:** Natural humectant (attracts moisture to hair) that also makes product thicker. Propylene glycol (a cheap, mineral oil-based substitute) is often used in formulas for the same purpose. **Wheat Protein:** Adds "substantivity" to hair, i.e., a thicker feel. Also helps coat hair shaft to repair damaged hair. **Aloe Vera:** All-around excellent hair and scalp treatment. **White Camellia Oil:** Traditionally used in Oriental countries, this oil is high in EFAs (essential fatty acids) that are moisturizing to the hair and skin. **Rosa Mosqueta®:** South American oil shown to have superb results with dry and damaged hair. **Macadamia Nut Oil:** Very moisturizing, without being greasy. **Almond Oil:** Excellent hair moisturizer. **Geranium, Lavender, Orange Blossom and Jasmine Oils:** Essential oils added for their calming and fragrant properties. **Rose Water:** Natural fragrance used for thousands of years as a soothing and moisturizing ingredient in hair and skin products. It was used by the physician, Galen, in ancient Egypt. **Natural Vitamin E Oil:** Added for its antioxidant properties, it protects oils from rancidity and helps preserve product. **Citrus Seed Extract and Vitamins A, C & E:** A natural preservative which protects both the oil and water phase of a product. Citrus and grapefruit seed extracts are currently being studied as treatments for yeast infections.

A synthetic shampoo label

Henna Shampoo for Blond Hair

Water, Henna Extract, Chamomile Extract, Sodium Olefin Sulfonate, Cocoamide DEA, Sodium Myeth Sulfate, TEA Lauryl Sulfate, Panthenol, Wheat Germ Oil, Hexadecanol, EGMS, Amodimethicone, Lemongrass Oil, Citrus Acid, Methylparaben, Germall, Fragrance.

Water: What kind of water? (Distilled is best.) **Henna Extract:** What is the strength of the extract? Is it extracted in water or something else? Is it neutral (i.e. noncoloring) henna? **Chamomile Extract:** How extracted? What strength? **Sodium Olefin Sulfonate:** Synthetic detergent. May be irritating and drying to hair and skin. **Cocoamide DEA:** Foam stabilizer and thickener. Synthetic. *DEA* stands for diethanolamine, which may be contaminated with nitrosamines. **Sodium Myeth Sulfate:** Synthetic detergent. Not biodegradable. May leave hair dry and dull. **TEA Lauryl Sulfate:** Synthetic detergent, stronger than above, combined with triethanolamine to balance the acidity of the shampoo and to thicken it. May be contaminated with nitrosamines. May be irritating to the skin. Drying to the hair. **Panthenol:** Provitamin B5, added to make hair feel thicker. **Wheat Germ Oil:** Rich in vitamin E, if protected with antioxidants, which it isn't; added for its moisturizing properties. **Hexadecanol:** Also known as cetyl alcohol. May be natural or synthetic. Added for its moisturizing properties. **Amodimethicone:** Silicone fluid used to give a smooth feel to product. May cause allergic reactions. **Lemongrass Oil:** Herbal, probably added for fragrance. **Citrus Acid:** Used as preservative, and an acidifier. **Methylparaben:** Synthetic preservative. Incompatible with protein and anionic surfactants, including TEA lauryl sulfate. **Germall:** Trade name for imidazolidinyl urea, a synthetic preservative that can release formaldehyde at over 10° C. **Fragrance:** What is this? May be natural or synthetic. Consumers need to know; fragrance is the leading cause of allergic reactions.

natural moisturizer label

ͺueta® Rose Hip Moisturizing Cream

Fatty Acid Cream Base, Aloe Vera, Rosa Mosqueta® Rose Hip Seed Oil, Horsetail, Coltsfoot, Nettle, Coneflower, St. John's Wort, Calendula, Sweet Almond Oil, Citrus Seed Extract with Vitamins A, C & E as preservative.

Fatty Acid Cream Base: This is used as a carrying agent and an absorption agent for the herbs and essential oils in the product. It is a natural ingredient made with coconut fatty acids. **Aloe Vera:** This is the liquid "gel" from the aloe vera plant. It is excellent for the skin as a moisturizer. **Rosa Mosqueta® Rose Hip Seed Oil:** A trade name for the oil obtained from the South American rose hip, which is the red seeds from the wild rose that grows in the Andes mountains *(Rosa aff. rubiginosa)*. The oil from these seeds is high in fatty acids and vitamin C. It is soothing and moisturizing to the skin, and known for its ability to reduce lines on the skin and help burns. **Horsetail:** This herb is excellent for the hair and skin. It is high in silica (7%), sulfur and fatty acid esters, which are texturizers and moisturizers to skin and hair. **Coltsfoot:** This herb is high in silica as well as amino acids such as cysteine, which are important to the hair and skin. **Nettle:** This herb has phytosterols which have been found to be excellent treatments for the skin and hair. It's said to stimulate hair growth by herbalists and is a mild skin astringent. It's high in protein, amino acids, and vitamins. **Coneflower:** This herb is an excellent skin soother and is so mild and healing it's been used in France as an eyewash since ancient times. **St. John's Wort:** This herbal extract is soothing to the skin. Excellent for sensitive skin. **Calendula:** *Calendula officinalis,* better known as marigold, is soothing to the skin. **Sweet Almond Oil:** Well known as a skin emollient. **Citrus Seed Extract with Vitamins A, C & E:** Used as a preservative.

A synthetic moisturizer label

Oil-Free Herbal Moisturizer

Infusions of Calendula, Cucumber, Echinacea, Suma, Aloe, Chamomile, Ginkgo Biloba, Rose Hips, Nettle and Geranium, Propylene Glycol, Glyceryl Stearate S. E., Octyl Hydroxystearate, Starch Octyl Succinate, Cetyl Alcohol, Polysorbate 40, Cyclomethicone, Hyaluronic Acid, NaPCA, Panthenol, Tetrasodium EDTA, Carbomer 940, Methylparaben, Propylparaben, Imidazolidinyl Urea, Fragrance (Essence Oil).

Infusions of Calendula, Cucumber, Echinacea, Suma, Aloe, Chamomile, Ginkgo Biloba, Rose Hips, Nettle and Geranium: This sounds good but tells us little. First, what is the strength of the infusion? 1%? 3%? With what kind of water? Distilled is best because it's purest. **Propylene Glycol:** Cheap synthetic humectant made from mineral oil. Choose vegetable glycerine instead. **Glyceryl Stearate S. E.:** Pearlizing agent, emulsifier, and opacifier. Synthetic. May cause irritation and clogged pores. **Octyl Hydroxystearate:** Fatty acid ester, an emollient and emulsifier. Synthetic. Possible irritant, allergic reactions. **Starch Octyl Succinate:** Thickener. **Cetyl Alcohol:** Fatty alcohol that may be natural or synthetic. Thickener and emollient. **Polysorbate 40:** Fatty acid ester used as emulsifier. May dry skin. **Cyclomethicone:** Added to give "smooth feel"—may cause allergic reactions. **Hyaluronic Acid:** Animal extract used as humectant. Panthenol or aloe vera mucopolysaccharide is just as effective, without harming animals. **NaPCA:** Synthetic chemical. Humectant. **Panthenol:** Vitamin B5. Good humectant. **Tetrasodium EDTA:** Sequestering agent. May cause severe irritation. **Carbomer 940:** Synthetic emulsifier that can cause irritation. **Methylparaben:** Preservative. Ineffective in products containing protein. **Propylparaben:** Synthetic preservative. See above. **Imidazolidinyl Urea:** Synthetic preservative. May release formaldehyde over temperatures of 10° C (50° F). **Fragrance (Essence Oil):** What "essence" oil? Fragrance frequently causes allergic reactions.

Ingredients good, natural manufacturers use

Colors

Good, natural manufacturers add no synthetic colors to their products. In fact, they use no colors at all. The colors of their products are just whatever colors the ingredients impart to them.

Disinfectants

A good natural compounder depends on the disinfecting and antifungal qualities of herbals such as camphor, eucalyptus, allspice and menthol. These substances not only protect the product from microbial, bacterial and fungal invasion, they do the same for your hair and skin.

Emollients

Emollients act to lubricate and soften skin. The most effective ones are those that are closest to your skin's natural sebum. Over 20 years ago, I pioneered the use of herbal oils such as evening primrose oil and Rosa Mosqueta® oil, and essential fatty acids, as emollients.

Emulsifiers

Many cosmetic products are emulsions (homogenous combinations of oil and water). Emulsions can be made and kept stable in a variety of ways. "Shake well before using" is one way; the use of vegetable glycerine and alcohol is another. (Most emulsions are made by assembling the oil and water phases separately, and then, with the appropriate heating and cooling phases, combining them.)

Ingredients synthetic manufacturers use

Colors

Some cosmetic manufacturers who sell in health food stores no longer use synthetic colors, but the vast majority still do. Watch out for D&C and FD&C colors; they're often carcinogenic and always unnecessary.

Disinfectants

Because synthetic products don't contain essential oils, they're far more vulnerable to microbial, bacterial and fungal attack, and their manufacturers must use strong disinfectants like hydroquinoline bromide to protect them. (Sometimes these disinfectants kill more than microbes. Hexachlorophene, for example, killed and brain-damaged babies, until it was discontinued.)

Emollients

Mineral oil and its derivatives are the substances most commonly used by synthetic manufacturers as emollients. They're photosensitizing, are absorbed poorly into the skin and, by interfering with the skin's natural moisturizing factor, actually produce dry skin. Most synthetic chemists don't see any difference between mineral oil and herbal oils. Petrolatum and glycerol stearate are two ingredients to avoid.

Emulsifiers

Surfactants (also known as surface-active agents) like propylene glycol, triethanolamine and hydroxymethyl cellulose are often used as emulsifiers by synthetic manufacturers. These chemicals can cause allergic reactions.

Ingredients good, natural manufacturers use

Essential oils

Herbal oils possess all kinds of therapeutic properties, both mentally and physically, but only when they're used in all-natural formulas. Some of the essential oils most commonly used are eucalyptus, camphor, menthol, camomile, balsam tolu, allspice, geranium, magnolia and Chinese herbals.

Gums

Herbal gums like gum tragacanth and gum arabic can be used to provide lift and body in hair gels, natural hair sprays and other hair-styling products. They work without drying your hair or adding petrochemicals to your body or the earth. They can also be combined with panthenol, a hair humectant and thickener.

Humectants

These ingredients, which attract water to skin and hold moisture in cosmetics, can also have a soothing effect on skin and hair. Natural humectants include vegetable glycerine, panthenol (vitamin B_5) and vitamin E.

Hair conditioners

Many natural substances can improve the feel and manageability of damaged hair, including proteins such as lactalbumin (from milk) and glycogen (from oysters), and sulphur-containing amino acids such as cysteine and methionine. Among the herbals long known for their hair-conditioning properties are rosemary, sage, balsam, horsetail and coltsfoot.

Ingredients synthetic manufacturers use

Fragrances

Because they were specifically exempted from the Label Reading Act of 1977, specific fragrances don't have to be listed as ingredients on bodycare products. Chances are if you see "fragrance" on a label, it's a synthetic chemical and not an essential oil.

Gums & PVP/VA copolymers

These chemicals are what most cosmetic manufacturers use in their hair-styling products. Typically combined with alcohol, synthetic emollients and synthetic preservatives, they're plastic films that coat your hair.

Humectants

The most commonly used synthetic humectant is propylene glycol, a mineral oil derivative. It's often combined with fatty acids, which may be either natural or synthetic, but in either case, the resulting compound can't be considered natural.

Hair conditioners

Quaternary ammonium compounds, chemicals originally developed as fabric softeners, are most commonly used as synthetic hair conditioners. They're quite toxic, and do nothing for the long-term health of your hair.

Ingredients good, natural manufacturers use

Soaps

Soaps are compounds that can dissolve in both oil and water. Made from fats, either animal or vegetable, and salts (such as lye or sea salt), they're more biodegradable than detergents. Vegetable soaps are also milder than detergents, but they may not work well in hard water if improperly formulated. With the use of various herbs and a skillful formula, hard water poses no problems, even for a totally natural soap.

Coconut oil soap is a mild cleanser made by naturally combining coconut oil and sea salt. It may be thickened with aloe vera. Olive oil, or castile, soap is another mild, vegetarian soap. Wheat or soy protein is a natural ingredient that helps build lather and condition hair.

Ingredients synthetic manufacturers use

Soaps and detergents

Synthetic manufacturers of cosmetics make their shampoos, facial cleansers and soap cakes with synthetic detergents (syndets). Syndets are similar to soap in that they can dissolve in both oil and water, but they aren't natural, and do the same kind of harm to our environment that laundry and household detergents do. (Though we usually don't think of shampoo polluting our water the way household cleansers do, it does.)

Syndets are made from a variety of petrochemicals that are far less biodegradable than soap and far less gentle on the skin. Many cosmetic manufacturers claim that sodium lauryl sulfate, and other syndets, come from coconuts. They do not—they're made by the Ziegler process with sulfur trioxide or chlorosulfuric acid.

Syndets are often combined with diethanolamine (DEA) or triethanolamine (TEA), either of which can form carcinogenic nitrosamines in hair care and skin care products. Here are some synthetic ingredients you should avoid in any cosmetics you buy:

- cocamide DEA
- cocamidopropyl betaine
- sodium laureth sulfate
- sodium lauryl sulfate
- TEA-lauryl sulfate

Ingredients good, natural manufacturers use

Preservatives

In 1973, Dr. Jakob Harich developed a preservative using grapefruit seed extract. He suggested I include it as an ingredient in my own preservative formula, which consisted of the antioxidant vitamins A, C and E.

This new natural preservative has proven to be both safe and effective, allowing products to be protected for a year or more. In fact, Dr. Harich's preservative can replace antibiotics that are widely used to feed farm animals.

Many essential oils, and other herbal extracts like benzoin gum, can protect products from spoiling. Look for these natural preservatives on cosmetic labels.

Ingredients synthetic manufacturers use

Preservatives

Most cosmetics are made in large batches and are mass-distributed; many are even shipped overseas. Because their synthetic chemical mix is vulnerable to microbial, bacterial and fungal contamination, these products need strong preservatives, and sometimes you'll see as many as five of them on a single label. Remember that they're put in to protect the manufacturers and their method of making products—not to protect you.

The most commonly used synthetic cosmetic preservatives are methyl and propyl paraben, which are strong sensitizers and can cause contact dermatitis. Formaldehyde is sometimes also used, in the form of DMDM Hydantoin. Other preservatives to avoid are imidazolidinyl urea, also sold under the trade name of Germall, and phenoxyethanol (a phenolic compound).

pH Balanced

On cosmetic labels, "pH-balanced" is another way to keep the attention of the consumer away from "the juice in the bottle." The pH of water is 7.0—perfectly neutral. The pH of the skin ranges from 4.0 to 6.75. The pH of bodycare products should be from 4.5 to 8, but why manipulate it with chemicals? After all, the pH of lemon juice and muriatic acid is both 2, but which would you rather put on your skin or hair?

Chapter 4
A natural method of skin and hair care

The following step-by-step diagrams will put you on the road to taking care of your complexion and your hair. I came up with this natural method of skin and hair care over twenty years ago, and first published it in the 1980s. Since then I've had the opportunity to refine and improve on it. I've found that women and men who put this system to work see remarkable changes in their skin and hair. (It is, however, only as good as the products you use.)

My natural method of skin care consists of seven steps. It's followed by an eleven-step massage that has been successful in combination with the skin care method. It's best to give yourself the massage right after you steam your skin. (If you don't happen to steam your skin, then do it when you apply a moisturizer.) Practice the massage diagrams until they're second nature and you'll be delighted with the results.

The final section of this chapter shows you the natural method of hair care I learned from my mother and that I've used for many years myself. It consists of just four steps, but people who use it tell me, "this saved my hair." I don't place much stock in "miracle hair growers," but the method I present here will do more than any "miracle product." Try it and find out for yourself.

Overview of natural method of skin care

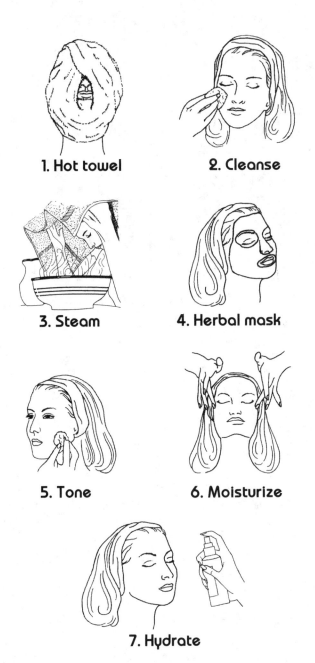

1. Hot towel

2. Cleanse

3. Steam

4. Herbal mask

5. Tone

6. Moisturize

7. Hydrate

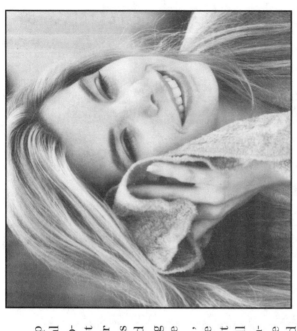

Step 1 · Soften and relax tissues

Before beginning your facial, remove all your makeup with a natural oil (jojoba, for example) or with a natural beauty oil that doesn't contain mineral oil or other petro-chemicals. Have a clean, hot towel ready, and some hot water to dampen it with. Wrap the hot towel around your face and leave it there until it begins to cool down. This first step will soften and relax tissues, open follicles and allow deep cleansing of the skin. As surface cells are softened, dead skin will be removed. This hot towel treatment will also increase circula-tion and will help the sweat glands get rid of toxins.

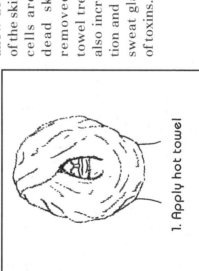

1. Apply hot towel

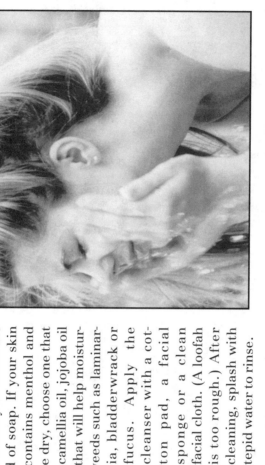

Step 2 · Cleanse your skin

After you remove the towel, you're ready to clean the skin. Use a facial cleanser instead of soap. If your skin tends to be oily, choose one that contains menthol and peppermint. If your skin tends to be dry, choose one that contains herbal oils—such as white camellia oil, jojoba oil or Rosa Mosqueta® (rose hip) oil—that will help moisturize your skin, or moisturizing seaweeds such as laminaria, bladderwrack or fucus. Apply the cleanser with a cotton pad, a facial sponge or a clean facial cloth. (A loofah is too rough.) After cleaning, splash with tepid water to rinse.

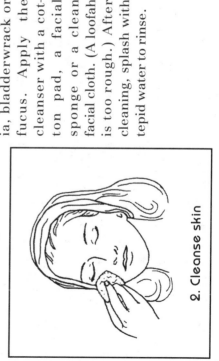

2. Cleanse skin

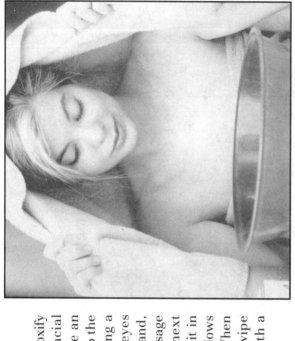

Step 3 · Steam and massage

Applying steam to the face is an excellent way to detoxify and deep-cleanse your skin. If you don't have a facial steamer, you can use a bowl of boiling water. Place an herbal tea into the steamer, or a handful of herbs into the boiling water. Place a towel over your head, creating a "tent," with your face close to the steam and your eyes closed. Apply some natural herbal oil to your hands and, following the massage diagrams in the next section, massage it in while the steam flows over your skin. When you're through, wipe the oils away with a damp cloth.

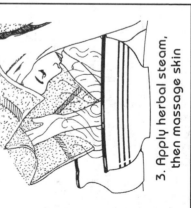

3. Apply herbal steam, then massage skin

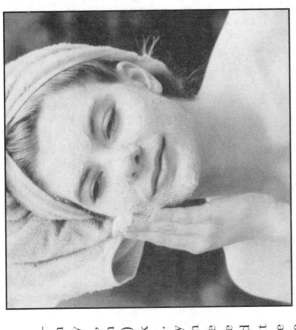

Step 4 · Apply an herbal mask

Facial masks deep-cleanse the skin by drawing out impurities and encouraging rapid turnover of old skin cells with new and healthier ones. You can make your own mask by blending herbs into carrying and binding agents like eggs, honey, yogurt and buttermilk. Or you can purchase an herbal facial mask (or the ingredients to make your own) at a health food store. You can alternate the herbal mask with a fruit acid mask.

Clay masks usually shouldn't be used on skin that tends to be too dry. Apply the mask once a week and leave it on for about ten minutes. Remove it by washing it off. Be careful not to get the mask in your eyes.

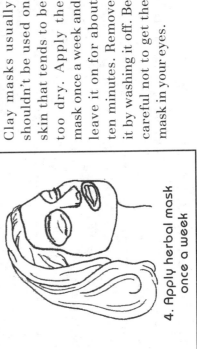

4. Apply herbal mask once a week

297

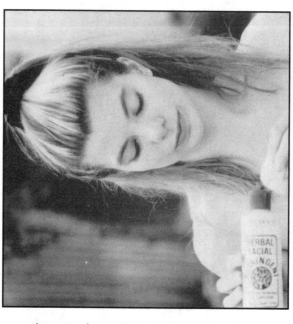

Step 5 · Toning the skin

The purpose of this step, which is sometimes called "clearing" the skin, is to prepare the skin for moisturization. Astringents are important to your skin, but quite often they are manufactured with acetone, alcohol and petrochemicals, which are hardly what you want to put on the skin as a method of "clearing" and toning it. Choose a pure herbal astringent that contains witch hazel and no more than 15% alcohol. Apply the astringent to a cotton ball and wipe the skin with an upward and outward motion.

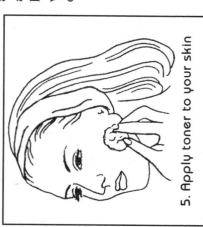

5. Apply toner to your skin

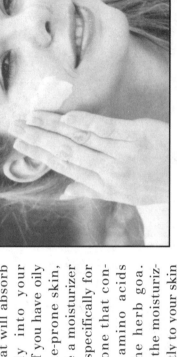

Step 6 · Moisturizing the skin

This step is only difficult because of the many moisturizers for sale and the claims made for them (everything from making you young again to taking away all your wrinkles). Ignore the hype and look at the ingredients instead. You want a moisturizer that has a natural base made with fatty acids—a light cream that will absorb quickly into your skin. If you have oily or acne-prone skin, choose a moisturizer made specifically for that, one that contains amino acids and the herb goa. Apply the moisturizer lightly to your skin (don't use too much).

6. Apply moisturizer and massage gently into skin

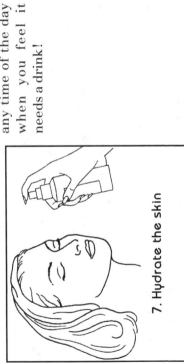

Step 7 · Hydrate the skin

This last step seems so simple—all you do is apply an herbal, mineral water spray to your skin. You can obtain the spray at a health food store or make your own (just add an herbal tea that's good for the skin, and perhaps some vitamins, to sparkling mineral water). Spray the store-bought or home-made mineral water mixture lightly over the moisturizer you applied in Step 6.

You can also hydrate your skin at other times as well—any time of the day when you feel it needs a drink!

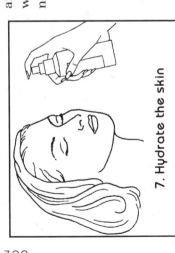

7. Hydrate the skin

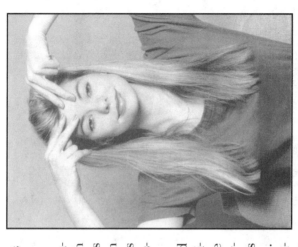

Step 1 · Circular massage of the forehead

To begin, pour a small pool of a completely natural beauty oil (made with herbal extracts or mild essential oils only) into your palms and rub them together. This gives "slip" to the hands during the massage, and lightly moisturizes the skin.

For Step 1, move the middle and index fingers of both hands in a semicircular movement. Beginning on the right temple (see the * in the drawing), apply light, circular strokes (called effleurage) to the left temple. Then do the same from the left temple to the right. Don't lift your fingers; the movement should be smooth and even—a steady, fluid motion. Repeat this five times.

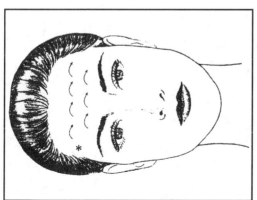

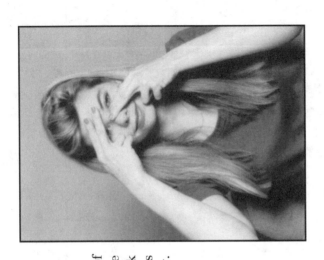

Step 2
Criss-cross massage
of the forehead

Using the middle and index fingers of both hands, begin at the left temple (at the * in the drawing) and work from left to right, using criss-cross motions. Finish by pressing lightly. Repeat this five times.

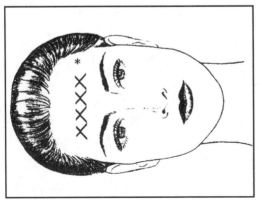

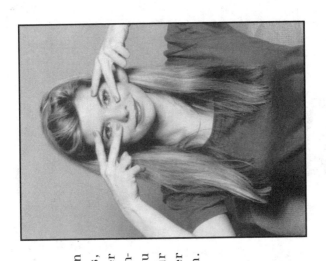

Step 3
Eye area massage

Using a very gentle touch on the thin and delicate skin around the eyes, place the middle fingers at the inner corners of the eyes and the index fingers over the brows (almost as if you were forming a mask around your eyes). Slide the fingers to the outer corner of the eyes and back again. Repeat this five times.

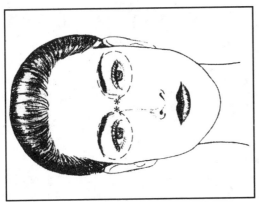

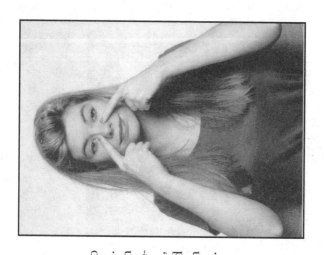

Step 4
Massage of
the nose area

Slide your fingers from the eye area to each side of the bridge of the nose. Press firmly and rotate once, then slide down the nose in a circular movement (effleurage). Press and rotate, press and rotate. End by pressing and rotating on the tip of your nose, then return to the beginning position. Repeat this three times.

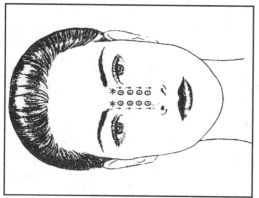

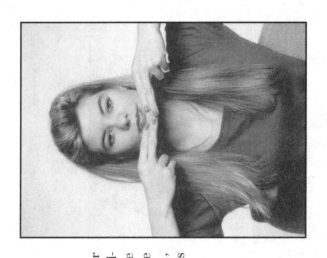

Step 5
Massage around the mouth

Slide your right hand under your chin, and bring the thumb and middle finger up to the corners of the mouth. Do a circular effleurage five times. Continue around the mouth, pressing and rotating. Repeat this three times.

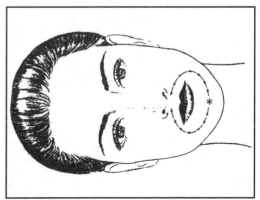

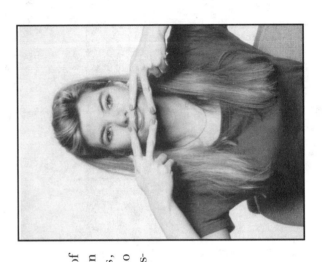

Step 6
Massage the cheeks

Using the middle and index fingers of both hands, massage from the chin across the cheeks to the earlobes, and from the corners of the nose to the tips of the ears. Repeat this massage five times.

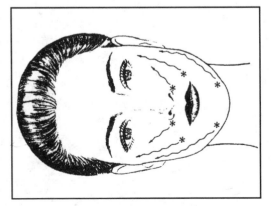

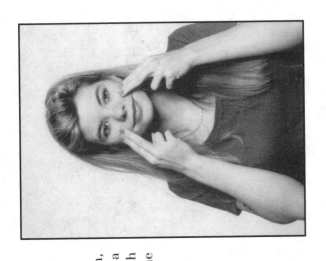

Step 7
Pressing massage of the cheeks

Beginning at the corners of the mouth, gently but firmly tap the face with a lifting and dropping motion of both hands (do both sides of the face at the same time). Repeat this five times.

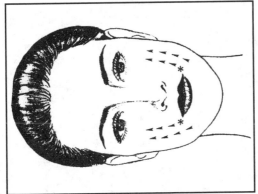

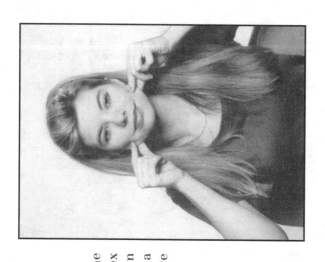

Step 8
Massage the sides of the face

Grasp the flesh of the chin with the thumb and the knuckle of the index finger of both hands. Work up, then down, both sides of the face with a plucking movement. Repeat this five times.

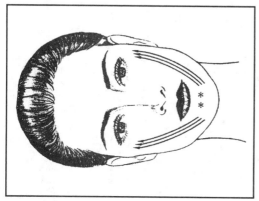

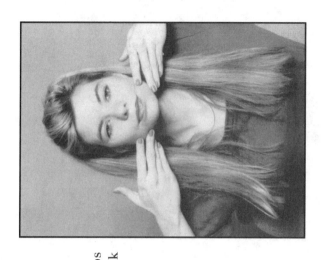

Step 9
Massage under
the jaw line

Gently lift the jaw line with the tips of the fingers and slide it back toward the ears.

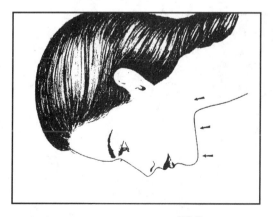

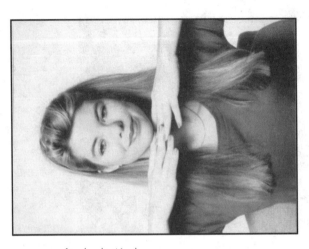

Step 10
Massage under the jaw

Place both hands palms down under your neck, with your fingertips intertwined. Keeping the fingertips together, begin a scissor-like movement back and forth. Repeat this movement five times.

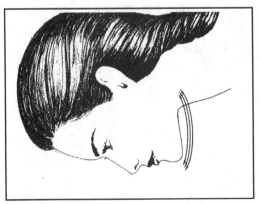

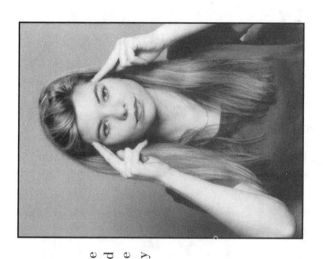

Step 11
Completing the facial massage

To complete the facial massage, place your fingertips on your temples and gently rotate. Then press for three seconds. Repeat five times, gradually tapering off the pressure

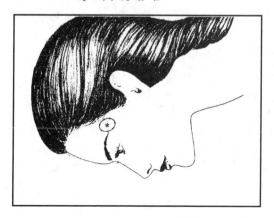

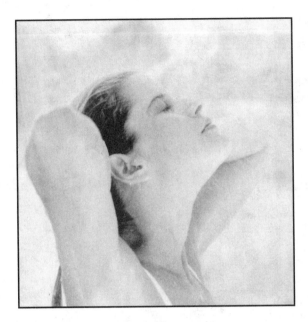

Step 1 · Shampoo your hair

The idea that the hair is "dead fabric" is absurd, because it and the scalp are able to absorb substances that not only change the hair but our health in general. Here are some suggestions for choosing a shampoo for your hair type.

Normal to oily hair: Look for essential oils and herbals like quillaya bark (which helps clean the hair without adding oils) and amino acids mixed with saponins (which help oily scalps become less oily). Non-coloring henna and peppermint are also excellent for oily hair. Change shampoos from time to time.

Normal to dry hair: Look for essential oils and herbals that add extra conditioning, such as jojoba oil, Rosa Mosqueta® oil, evening primrose oil, blue camomile oil, white camellia oil and the B vitamin panthenol.

Damaged hair & hair loss: Dry, brittle hair, and hair that's been "salon-damaged" by coloring, permanents or straighteners can benefit from sulfur-containing amino acids. Look on the label for the herbs horsetail and colts-foot, and for the amino acid cysteine.

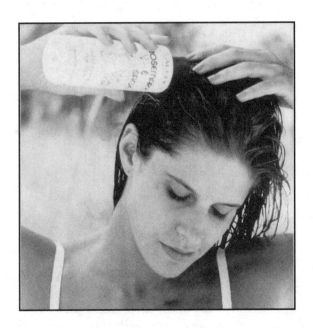

Step 2 · Herbal rinse for your hair

After you've rinsed the shampoo out with warm water, apply an herbal rinse to your hair. This will "clear" the hair, much as an astringent "clears" the skin.

Normal to oily hair: If your hair tends to be oily, look for an herbal rinse with peppermint and noncoloring henna in it. You can also make a rinse by boiling rosemary, sage and peppermint tea with lemon peels. For oily hair, you should apply a conditioner (see Step 3) *first,* then use the herbal rinse.

Normal to dry hair: You can look for the herbals listed in the previous paragraph, but in addition to using the rinse, you should give your hair a "hot oil treatment" with any of the following oils: jojoba, Rosa Mosqueta® or evening primrose. Heat the oil and work it through your hair about 15 to 20 minutes before you wash it.

Damaged hair & hair loss: Also use a "hot oil treatment," as described in the previous paragraph.

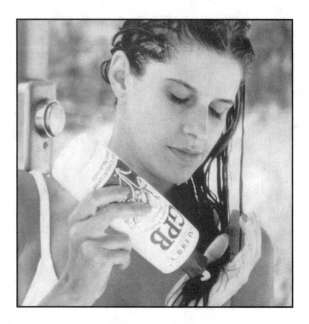

Step 3 · Condition your hair

Applying a good natural conditioner to your hair is an important step for all hair types. Here are my suggestions:

Normal to oily hair: Look for hair conditioners with milk proteins such as lactalbumin, the herbs horsetail and coltsfoot, and the amino acid cysteine. As mentioned above, apply this conditioner first, *then* apply the herbal rinse (Step 2).

Normal to dry hair: In addition to horsetail and coltsfoot, aloe vera and jojoba oil are very helpful to dry hair. Also look for shea butter, evening primrose oil and Rosa Mosqueta® oil. You should give your hair a "hot oil treatment," as described under *Normal to dry hair* in Step 2.

Damaged hair & hair loss: Use the treatment described in the previous paragraph. The B vitamin panthenol will also help (see Step 4 for more about it).

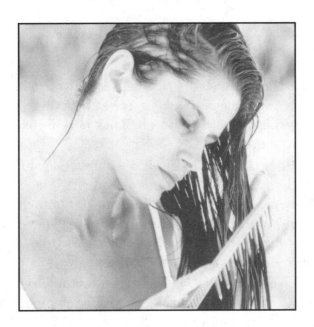

Step 4 · Style your hair

Applying a synthetic styling gel, hairspray or hairset often dries out the hair, making it brittle and "straw-like." Instead, use natural products with the following ingredients:

You want **a hairspray** that contains gum arabic, gum tragancanth and panthenol. In additon to helping the holding action of the herbal gums, panthenol adds thickness to the hair, making it look fuller, and it's a great moisturizer as well. (Once, when I removed the lid from a jar of panthenol I had on the shelf in my lab, I found beads of moisture inside the lid.) I've used panthenol with great success in hair and skin care.

A styling gel should contain Rosa Mosqueta® oil or white camellia oil, as well as gum arabic, gum tragancanth and panthenol.

A "luster" or "shine" spray should also contain Rosa Mosqueta® oil or white camellia oil. It should make the hair shiny and reduce tangles and snarls, and it shouldn't be greasy or oily.

About the author

Aubrey Hampton was born on an organic farm in rural Indiana and educated in New York City. At the age of nine, he began learning how to make herbal cosmetics from his mother.

In 1967, Hampton founded Aubrey Organics®, a natural and organic cosmetics company. Since then, he has created and marketed over 200 natural hair, skin and bodycare products. Virtually every health food store in the United States carries them, as do many in Europe, Asia and elsewhere.

A phytochemist and herbalist, Hampton gives seminars throughout the world in which he demonstrates how cosmetics can be made completely naturally, without harming the environment, and without being tested on animals. In 1990, the Culture and Animals Foundation named him Activist of the Year for his work promoting animal rights and the environment.

In 1969, Hampton began publishing *Organic World Newsletter.* A year later, he brought out the first issue of *Organica Quarterly;* it's still being published, and now has more than 100,000 readers.

In 1990, Hampton's biographical drama about George Bernard Shaw, *GBS & Company,* was nominated for the Bernard Hewitt Award and the George Freedley Memorial Award. Colin Wilson called the play "a splendid piece of work" and wrote that "Aubrey Hampton knows Shaw as well as Shaw knew Shakespeare."

In 1991, Hampton published *Wolf Trilogy.* According to Victoria Moran, this play shows, "without preaching, [how] the much-maligned wolf paral-

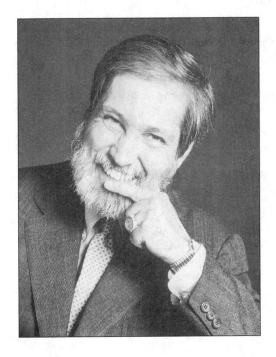

lels our own lives—a valuable message for the environmental decade and the future of all life."

Hampton's play, *Mixed Blood: A Drama about the Creation of the AIDS Virus* (1990), garnered praise from critics nationwide. *The New York Native* described it as "perhaps the first and only play to challenge the conventional wisdom about AIDS," and *The Oregonian* called it "a chilling drama theorizing how the AIDS epidemic began."

What's in Your Cosmetics? is Aubrey Hampton's first book for Odonian Press. His earlier book on the same subject, *Natural Organic Hair and Skin Care,* which he self-published, has sold more than 200,000 copies.

We also publish the Real Story series. It's based on a simple idea:

What Uncle Sam Really Wants   **Noam Chomsky**

A brilliant overview of the real motivations behind US foreign policy, from the man the *New York Times* called "arguably the most important intellectual alive." Chomsky's most popular book, it's full of astounding information. *111 pp. $5.* "Highly recommended." *—Booklist*

> **69,000 copies in print**

The Prosperous Few & the Restless Many   **Noam Chomsky**

A wide-ranging report that covers everything from Bosnia to NAFTA. Chomsky's fastest-selling book ever, it was on the *Village Voice Literary Supplement's* best-sellers list for six months running. *95 pp. $5.* "Calmly reasoned. Most welcome." *—Newsday*

> **54,000 copies in print**

Secrets, Lies and Democracy   **Noam Chomsky**

The latest in Chomsky's series of state-of-the-world reports, this fascinating volume concludes with a list of 144 organizations worth putting time and effort into. *127 pp. $6.*

The Chomsky Trilogy   **Noam Chomsky**

The three books listed above, in a handsome boxed set. *$15.*

The CIA's Greatest Hits   **Mark Zepezauer**

In crisply written, two-page chapters, each accompanied by a cartoon, this book describes the CIA's many attempts to assassinate democracy all over the world. *95 pp. $6.*

Burma: The Next Killing Fields?   **Alan Clements**

If we don't do something about Burma, it will become another Cambodia. Written by one of the few Westerners ever to have lived there, this book tells the story vividly. *95 pp. $5.* "Deserves to be in every library." *—Library Journal*

Our books are available at discriminating bookstores everywhere. But if, through some fluke, you can't find them, you can also buy them directly from us—Odonian Press, Box 32375, Tucson AZ 85751. ⇨   ⇨   ⇨

Political books don't have to be boring.

The Decline and Fall of the American Empire   **Gore Vidal**
Gore Vidal is one of our most important—and wittiest—social critics. This delightful little book is the perfect introduction to his political views. *95 pp. $5.* "*Acerbic, deliciously, maliciously funny.*"—New York Times Book Review

The Greenpeace Guide to
** Anti-environmental Organizations**   **Carl Deal**
A comprehensive guide to more than 50 industry front groups that masquerade as environmental organizations. The deception is amazing. *110 pp. $5.* "*Fascinating. A must.*" —New Orleans Times-Picayune

Who Killed JFK?   **Carl Oglesby**
"I'm just the patsy," said Lee Harvey Oswald, and truer words were never spoken. This fact-filled guide gives you the inside story on the most famous crime of the twentieth century. *95 pp. $5.* "*A must-have for all serious students of the assassination.*" —Midwest Book Review

Who Killed Robert Kennedy?   **Philip Melanson**
This carefully researched book explains why Sirhan *couldn't* have murdered RFK, and discusses who the actual killers might have been. *94 pp. $5.* "*Persuasive.*" —Publishers Weekly

Who Killed Martin Luther King?   **Philip Melanson**
This fascinating investigation of a murder that changed history shows why the official story—that James Earl Ray did it—just doesn't hold water. *94 pp. $5.* "*Concise. Hardhitting.*" —Oliver Stone

Our shipping charge is just $2 per order, regardless of the number of books. (If you're an Arizona resident, please add 7% tax.) To order by credit card, or for information on quantity discounts, call us at 520 296 4056 or 800 REAL STORY, or fax us at 520 296 0936.

Also available from Odonian Press:

With well over a hundred million users, coffee is far and away the most popular drug in the United States (alcohol is second, tobacco third, marijuana fourth).

Virtually everyone who drinks it wonders if coffee has any harmful side effects but, amazingly, this is the *only* popular overview of the extensive research that's been done on the subject.

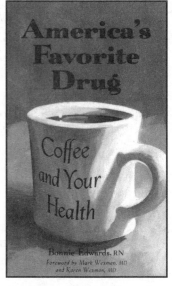

In just 111 pages, this easy-to-read, $5 guide tells you everything that's known about the health effects of coffee. It covers cholesterol, blood pressure, heart problems, cancer, fibrocystic breasts, infertility, pregnancy, breast feeding, PMS, digestive disorders, sleep disturbance, lung function, headaches, vision changes, vitamin and mineral depletion, anxiety and panic attacks, and intensification of tobacco withdrawal symptoms. (Not all the news is bad, by the way.)

There's a discussion of other chemicals besides caffeine that are found in coffee. Various decaffeination methods are compared, as is the caffeine content of coffee, teas and colas. Most chapters end with a section called *What you can do,* and the discussion of coffee withdrawal symptoms includes recommended strategies for quitting or cutting down.

If you drink coffee, you owe it to yourself to check out *America's Favorite Drug: Coffee and Your Health.*